Stress Free Pregnancy

Stress Free Pregnancy

108 Essential Tips for Enjoying a Peaceful Pregnancy

TARA BIANCA

one love heals all

This publication contains the opinions and ideas of the author. It is intended to provide helpful and informative material on the subjects addressed in the publication. It is sold with the understanding that the author and publisher are not engaged in rendering medical, health, psychological or any other kind of personal professional services in the book. If the reader requires personal medical, health or other assistance or advice a competent professional should be consulted.

Although the author and publisher have made every effort to ensure that the information in this book is accurate and current, only your caregiver knows you and your health history well enough to make specific recommendations. The authors, editors, reviewers, and publisher disclaim any liability, loss or risk, personal or otherwise, that is incurred as a consequence, directly or indirectly of the use and application of the contents of this book.

Stress Free Pregnancy:
108 Essential Tips for Enjoying a Peaceful Pregnancy

Published by OneLoveHealsAll Publishing

ISBN: 978-0-9920161-0-4

Printed in the USA

Cover photo by © Alex Bramwell | Dreamstime.com
Author photo by Melissa Skoda
Illustrations by Mark Siermaczeski | Crueltyfreecartoons.com

Dedicated to the children of the future

and my beautiful baby Kai

Contents

Inspirational Reflections

All stress begins with one negative thought. ~ *Ben Johnson*

Stress is basically a disconnection from the earth, a forgetting of the breath.
Stress is an ignorant state. It believes that everything is an emergency.
Nothing is that important. Just lie down. ~ *Natalie Goldberg*

You always do what you want to do. This is true with every act. You may say that you had
to do something, or that you were forced to, but actually, whatever you do, you do by choice.
Only you have the power to choose for yourself. ~ *W. Clement Stone*

The wisdom and compassion a woman can intuitively experience in childbirth can make her
a source of healing and understanding for other women. ~ *Stephen Gaskin*

...celebrate ourselves for our courage to birth. The real question becomes not, 'Have you
done your breathing exercises?' but rather, 'Can you love yourself no matter how you birth,
where you birth, or what the outcome?' ~ *Claudia Panuthos*

1

Introduction

The mind that is anxious about future events is miserable.

~*Seneca*

A peaceful pregnancy is not found, it is consciously chosen and experienced. Ultimately, you are the only one who can create a peaceful, stress free environment for you and your baby. It is about embracing the freedom to make the choice to enjoy a peaceful, joyful, balanced prenatal experience. A beautiful opportunity is available if you are willing to dive into unconditional love for yourself and your baby, to embrace the knowing that you are worth the peace, and to transcend the limiting beliefs and even patterns of behavior that keep you fearful and small. It is allowing and choosing the best of you.

I'm here to reveal to you that you deserve to enjoy a peaceful pregnancy. But there's a caveat to this revelation: to experience a stress free pregnancy you're going to have to take responsibility and choose it at a core level. You'll then need to follow the suggestions and utilize the strategies in this book. Taking responsibility is essential because no one but you can choose to create a peaceful pregnancy.

With everything you are experiencing and learning during your pregnancy, probably the last thing you want to hear is that you need to take more responsibility or do more, but you do. The good news is that taking responsibility is actually freeing. It is an opportunity to enjoy an amazingly peaceful pregnancy. You know what it feels like to experience joy and peace. The emotional and health benefits for you and your baby outweigh the steps to get there.

A stress free pregnancy is not about perfection or obsessing about doing everything 'right.' This book is an open invitation on enjoying a pregnancy free of stress, anxiety and overwhelm. It may directly call in to question why you are allowing yourself to live at the energetic level where you currently reside, and it will playfully challenge you to live a more peaceful, joyful and balanced pregnancy and life. The key to this book is to do the best you possibly can by educating yourself with the information within and by applying the helpful strategies offered.

Unfortunately, the world of pregnancy has become imbued with an over indulgence of women giving their power away to the medicalization of the birthing industry. Women's innate prenatal and birthing experiences in the US are treated as medical conditions. While sitting with women, I have heard the same story recounted of how anxious, stressed and worried pregnant women are. And those who can financially afford it, add to their own anxiety by mimicking the medical industry by buying home Dopplers or worrying that they need unnecessary medical tests. It's unnecessary that so many women's prenatal experiences are being hijacked by excessive worry and suffering.

Medical care associated with childbirth has changed drastically over the last 100 years. We have new technologies, information, pain management techniques and prenatal care. Despite the increase of medical intervention, access to health care, healthy options, and a huge drop in infant death, women are reporting high fear and anxiety levels around pregnancy and birthing. It is because of prenatal worry, anxiety and stress that I wanted to write a book to empower expecting women to create a beautiful prenatal experience.

If you are one of many women who experiences anxiety and stress during pregnancy or you would love to experience the best possible pregnancy or you may be lacking some crucial strategies for enjoying an amazing pregnancy, then this book is for you.

While it may be normal to experience stress, how you deal with it is a significant factor in the health and wellness of you and your baby. Throughout your pregnancy, chronic or intense stress can lead to a number of complications for both you and your child. Neuropsychiatrist Richard Restak, M.D., summarizes the research on stress in a simple way for everyone to understand: "Stress causes brain damage." Not only has long-term stress been shown in study after study to injure the brain, but it also has devastating effects on the rest of the body. These effects extend to the development of your baby's brain, nervous system and organs.

This book is designed to provide information and tools to transform and eliminate stress so your pregnancy is as peaceful and relaxing as it can be. It is designed to remind you that your pregnancy is a time to celebrate, to set aside the day-to-day worries and to enjoy your growing baby and the fullness of your prenatal experience.

In the following pages you will find a practical guide that informs, inspires and provides tools to experience nourishment and a new gentleness toward yourself. As I have written this book, I have thought about you and your baby. The pages are filled with helpful information on the effects of stress on both of you, as well as insightful quotes and easy to apply inspirational advice on how to shift a stressful state into a joyful experience. The strategies can be done by anyone, don't take much time from your day and will add a new richness to your life.

This book isn't only for an expecting mother. It is here for you and your partner to share so you can both navigate through your prenatal experiences together in a supportive and loving way. Whether this is your first pregnancy or your second, third or fourth, this book is designed to be a valuable resource that will help you enjoy each day until you hold your baby in your arms.

You have the power to transform your state of being and to enjoy your pregnancy. As you read this book may you find in its pages a calming influence that will lift your mind and spirit.

From my heart to yours,

Tara Bianca

What is Stress?

S tress is a common experience that can affect people of all ages at any time in life, even your unborn baby. Before we get into the many ways to make your pregnancy stress free, it may be helpful to gain a greater understanding of what stress is and the effects that stress has on your body and mind.

What is Stress?

Stress is a subjective term that is not easy to define since it is a unique and personal experience. It was initially defined by endocrinologist Hans Seyle as the "the non-specific response of the body to any demand for change."

When faced with unresolved outside pressures or internal worries, stress can accumulate and contribute to mental, physical and emotional patterns, imbalances and symptoms. For example, a typical response to stress can be constricted or shallow breathing that may result in stress to your major organs. The tightening of muscles can be another automatic stress response that contributes to a restriction of blood flow and energy in the body, which can lead to an array of physical problems.

The symptoms of stress are simply the body's way of responding to demands placed upon our body and mind. They are informing and providing you an opportunity to deal with and resolve the demands before they get out of hand. Ignoring stressful conditions will not improve the situation. Avoiding taking responsibility to resolve the issues that are affecting you will only complicate your life and create additional stress.

In more complex terms, stress is part of a system of chemical reactions that occurs when we have an experience that incites a strong emotional reaction. When you encounter a stressful situation, chemicals such as cortisol are released into the body as a survival reaction for increased strength and additional energy, which is beneficial in case of emergencies. The stress response, in this case, gives us exactly what we need to overcome a situation.

This stress is usually temporary. After the situation, your nervous system begins the process of shutting down the release of chemicals and calming your body. It can take a fair amount of time but eventually, the stress leaves your body and you are no longer in a state of readiness.

Types of Stress

Typically people think of stress as a negative response with physical, mental or emotional distress. However, some types of stress can be positive and helpful. Beyond negative and positive stressors, there are neutral stressors that can be defined as experiences that on their own are neither negative nor are they positive. Most stressors fall into the neutral category until our beliefs and thoughts change them into a negative or positive experience.

Eustress or Positive Stress

Eustress is positive type of stress that may give you the energy and focus you need to finish a project or avoid danger. Eustress is also helpful for making important changes in our life, problem solving and being more efficient. Eustress can be triggered by weddings, taking a vacation, buying a new home or finding out you are having a baby.

Eustress causes the release of chemicals such as dopamine, oxytocin, adrenalin and serotonin, which gives you a feeling of wellness and happiness. Short-term eustress can help build many positive traits such as confidence, feelings of peace and contentment. Even though eustress can be a positive stress, if you become chronically over stimulated by adrenaline and don't use it up, the body will begin to experience the excess adrenaline as negative stress. A few ways to ensure a balanced approach includes creating opportunities for fun and laughter, exercising, meditating, relaxing and choosing not to over-commit your self.

Distress or Negative Stress

Distress, on the other hand, is a negative stress that feels unpleasant, causes anxiety, decreases our performance, and leads to many physical, emotional, and mental health problems. Distress occurs when you have an experience or emotion that creates a fight or flight reaction.

Financial problems, trauma, injury, illness, relationship issues, legal problems, job insecurity and excess responsibilities are just some of the outside events that could potentially produce a negative stress reaction. Internal beliefs and expectations can also trigger distress. These include internal experiences such as perfectionist expectations, phobias and worries about the future. For some expecting women, the internal fear of being a new mom can cause distress.

When you experience distress, your body produces hormones and chemicals such as cortisol and adrenaline, which lead to bursts of energy and strength, but also lead to a crash once the situation is over. When negative stress is emotional, the body continues to produce the chemicals needed to deal with a life-threatening situation. However, your body is not using those chemicals. The chemical overload builds and each new worry or emotional experience that causes a stress reaction will just compound the problem. This can lead to many negative side effects for you and your baby.

Hyperstress

Hyperstress is a type of stress that occurs when a person experiences an overload of stress that creates a severe emotional response. It can occur when a person is faced with a task or responsibility that is outside of their normal capacity. Tight deadlines, heavy workloads or poor self esteem can lead to severe overwhelm that may result in procrastination, an emotional outburst, a breakdown or an inability to do anything.

Hypostress

In contrast to hyperstress, hypostress is experienced when a person feels bored, underwhelmed or unchallenged. The symptoms can include lack of energy, loss of creativity, agitation, depression or feeling restless simply because the person is not being challenged, their work is repetitive or they are under-stimulated. Although this may not sound like an issue, it can lead to other forms of stress and stress related health problems.

Sources of Stress

When we think of all of these stresses, we also need to look at the forces that influence stress in our life. These internal or external influences shape the type of stress that we experience. Some of the more common sources of stress are:

- *Survival Stress* - Under the category of acute distress, this is stress when you have a fight or flight situation. When you are in a physical situation where your life or body is in danger, the body naturally produces an adrenaline burst to give you the strength to fight or the energy for flight for survival. While distress has a negative effect on the body, in an emergency it is an important stress response because it can save your life.

- *Environmental Stress* - Distress that is caused by an external force is known as environmental stress. This is different for everyone but it can be things such as a crowded store, pressures at work, pollutants or family stress. Your body will do its best to respond to outside stress to regulate and create chemical and hormonal balance. However, too much distress will begin to show up with progressively worse symptoms until the source of stress is addressed.

- *Internal Stress* - This kind of stress encompasses inner conflict, emotional or mental thoughts of worry around things we cannot control and expectations that we place on ourselves. During a pregnancy it can show up as worry or anxiety about the health of the baby or about the upcoming months of pregnancy and the lifetime of motherhood. Internal worries can become a chronic stress that contributes to a less fulfilling pregnancy and can put unnecessary stress on you and the baby. Internal stress is different for each person. One woman may let her pregnancy unfold and find joy in the new experience by dealing with situations as an opportunity to learn and grow. Another woman may allow herself to worry about possible negative outcomes.

- *Physical Stress/Fatigue Stress* - Physical stress entails any influence that can affect the physical health of any part of your body: muscles, ligaments, bones, hormones, digestive system, organs and skin. Lifting beyond your ability, staying up too late, eating toxic foods and physical exhaustion from working too much and too long without breaks can contribute to physical or fatigue stress, especially when you are pregnant.

Symptoms & Effects of Stress

In most cases, you usually know when you are experiencing negative stress. However, people may overlook the first signs that they are stressed or have symptoms that they are not aware are related to stress. This can lead to chronic stress that is more challenging to resolve. I've included a partial list below of symptoms often associated with stress to assist you to have a broader view of potential stressors in your life.

Stress can affect you physically, mentally and emotionally in a multitude of ways. With the early stages of stress, symptoms can include nail biting, twitching, blinking, fatigue, difficulty falling asleep, an increased heartbeat, cold hands and feet, upset digestive system, headaches, feelings of frustration or anger, dry mouth, increased urination, feeling mildly depressed or anxious, shortness of breath, increased sweating and muscle spasms.

If stress is dealt with early, most of the symptoms will go away as your body starts to relax and stops being in a state of readiness. If early signs of stress are left to compound, they can lead to symptoms of long-term stress in the mind and body.

Mind

We often think of physical ailments as the first indication that we are feeling stressed. However, in many cases, mental and thought based symptoms are usually the indication that you are overstressed. Some indicators that we may be mentally stressed include the inability to focus, reduced ability to remember, anxiety attacks, mood swings, nervousness, chronic worry, sleep problems, fatigue and depression. Eventually, unresolved stress will lead to more intense versions of stress symptoms and behaviors such as severe anxiety, terror, social detachment, feelings of hopelessness, irrational fears, severe fatigue, binge eating, major changes in sleep patterns, obsessive compulsive disorders and substance abuse.

Body

Your brain will send signals to your body to let you know that it is overstressed. However, many people do not pay attention to the symptoms and ignore them until a physical problem occurs. The more intense physical effects of stress often occur after there have been earlier signs of stress. If you have physical indicators of stress, pay attention. It is strong evidence that you need to resolve what ever is at the root of your stress. Some of the symptoms can include loss of sex drive, intestinal and stomach problems such as irritable bowl syndrome, loss of appetite, heart problems, breathing problems, body pain and aches, obesity, skin disorders and a compromised immune system.

Stress & Your Pregnancy

*D*ue to the physiological and biochemical changes during pregnancy, expecting women can experience a wide range of stress from mild to extreme. Understanding the external and internal influences and effects of prenatal stress is the first step to being motivated and informed on how to effectively manage and resolve stress during pregnancy. Since the effects of excessive maternal stress can result in harmful consequences, enjoying a stress free pregnancy is important not only for you but also for the health and well-being of your baby.

If stressful situations are infrequent, the human body has the ability to process excessive levels of stress hormones without too much damage. However, if an expecting woman experiences frequent, chronic or acute levels of stress, the high level of stress hormones becomes unmanageable. This contributes to health problems for both mom and baby, as excess stress hormones pass through the umbilical cord and placenta to the fetus.

The fetus then becomes imprinted with chemical information that informs it about the stressful environment it is being born into. This can have a profound effect on how the baby's DNA expresses itself. In addition, the stress chemicals contribute to developmental delays and health issues, not only in the womb but also after birth.

Effects of Stress on Your Pregnancy

In addition to the physical, mental and emotional symptoms reviewed earlier, there are several serious prenatal complications and consequences to experiencing stress during pregnancy.

Miscarriage

The most tragic result of excessive maternal stress for expecting women is a miscarriage. There are numerous studies that link stress, specifically acute stress due to a traumatic event, with a greater risk of miscarrying. However, even chronic stress can lead to a higher risk of miscarriage. This is due to the production of stress hormones, specifically corticotrophin-releasing hormone.[1] Negative emotions such as guilt, fear, anxiety, depression and feeling overwhelmed increases the odds of a miscarriage, especially in the first 12 weeks of pregnancy compared to those whose experience is happy, relaxed or in control. In addition, major social difficulties, poor relationships with partners and isolation have also been cited to influence miscarriage. Eating fruits and vegetables and taking prenatal vitamins have been shown to reduce the odds of miscarriage by approximately 50%, especially vitamins and foods that contains folic acid.[2]

Preterm Birth

Preterm birth is very common in women who smoke, drink alcohol, use drugs, have poor nutrition, work long hours, have physically demanding work, are exposed to environmental toxins or are under a significant amount of stress. There is also an increased risk of preterm birth with women who have high levels of pregnancy-related anxiety.[3]

16

A premature baby is at a greater risk for behavioral, cognitive, hearing, visual, growth, respiratory, immunologic, central nervous system and gastrointestinal problems. In addition, the family can experience significant economic and emotional hardships with the premature arrival of their baby.

Maternal Infections

Since stress often lowers the body's immune system, the chance of getting a uterine infection increases greatly in stressed pregnant women. Bacterial vaginosis, characterized by off-white discharge from the vagina, is also associated with high levels of chronic stress during pregnancy. While most infections can be treated, some infections can become quite serious resulting in premature labor or even miscarriage.

Preeclampsia

Preeclampsia is a very serious condition that results in visual disturbances, headaches and swelling in your hands and face. It is also linked to high blood pressure and protein in the urine. Left untreated, preeclampsia can result in death of both the mother and fetus.

Current research indicates that increased oxidative stress is one of the main causes of preeclampsia. Oxidative stress is cellular damage caused by free radicals (unstable oxygen molecules) randomly bombarding the body's cells. In general there are many different substances and processes that can contribute to oxidative stress including cigarette smoke, chlorinated water (that you drink or swim in), dehydration, processed sugar, hydrogenated fats, excessive animal protein, preservatives, food colorings, food flavorings, periodontal infection, pesticides, pharmaceuticals, pollution, radiation exposure and stress hormones.

Although very little is known about how to prevent preeclampsia, there are some indications[4] that a diet rich in antioxidants (greens, veggies and fruits) and foods high in omega-3 essential fatty acids (EFAs), such as walnuts, salmon, sardines, krill oil, flax seeds, chia seed, hemp seed, broccoli and spinach, may reduce the risk of preeclampsia. In addition, lowering levels of prenatal stress are also important for maternal and fetal health.

Effects of Stress on Your Baby

The stress a fetus is exposed to during gestation can negatively impact their mental and physical development. Interestingly, research on humans and animals has revealed that prenatal stress adversely affects the health of not just the developing fetus, but also that of the next generation.[5]

Preterm Birth

Although a preterm birth is something that affects your pregnancy, preterm birth also has many side effects on the baby. Babies who are born early often have a lifetime of complications such as developmental delays, chronic lung disease, heart disease and learning disorders. In addition, babies born prematurely due to prenatal stress are more likely to have high blood pressure as adults. Lastly, preterm babies often have a higher infant mortality rate than those born at full term.

Low Birth Weight

Low birth weight has been linked to high levels of stress and maternal consumption of cigarettes, drugs and alcohol. Low birth weight is a risk factor for infant mortality, preterm birth and developmental disabilities.

Developmental Delays

Acute prenatal stress can disrupt fetal brain development and can also impair development, learning capabilities and motor performance throughout early childhood.

Mood Disorders

Research has shown that a fetus's exposure to prenatal stress increases emotionality, behavioural issues, anxiety, depression, anger problems, bipolar disorder and difficulty dealing with high stress levels throughout their childhood and into adult life. Chronic and acute exposure to stress hormones can cause the offspring to develop an altered, life-long hyper-activation of the neuroendocrine system that controls reactions to stress and regulates digestion, the immune system, mood, emotions, sexuality and hormones.

Attention Disorders

Studies have shown there is a significant association between prenatal stress and increased risk for Autistic Disorder, hypersensitivity to stress and attention deficit/hyperactivity disorder (ADHD).[6]

Weak Immune Systems

Stress experienced by a pregnant woman also impacts the immune system of the fetus in detrimental and permanent ways, impacting the infant's immunology across its life span, setting up conditions that put the infant at greater risk for illnesses and other conditions that affect their quality of life.

Reducing Stress-Related Symptoms

Diet has been shown to help lower a fetus's vulnerability to stress-related conditions and illness. One research team concluded that expecting moms who consume greater amounts of choline (a nutrient found in eggs) may help mitigate exposure to stress.[7] Other research has found that iron, zinc and folic acid are important nutrients that alter brain development. A balanced diet is essential to ensure all vitamins, minerals, healthy fats and proteins are accessible to mom and the developing fetus. Once baby is born, mothers needs to continue to eat healthy, whole foods to replenish nutrients that have been depleted during pregnancy, especially when breastfeeding.

It is interesting to note that research also suggests that after delivery, mothers who stroke their newborn's body in the first month of their life could reverse some of the effects of prenatal stress.[8] Oxytocin, a hormone released during touch, has a role in healing, bonding, reducing anxiety, improving brain function, decreasing stress and producing feelings of calmness. A recent study revealed that oxytocin has also been found to improve the brain function of autistic children.[9] I was intrigued during my research to read one women's personal account of how constantly holding and breastfeeding her baby for six years resulted in what she believes may have been a reversal of autism.[10]

Causes of Stress During Pregnancy

How we perceive a situation and how we react to it is the basis of our stress. If you focus on the negative in any situation, you can expect high stress levels. However, if you try and see the good in the situation, your stress levels will greatly diminish.

~ *Catherine Pulsifer*

Although stress may seem like it is externally driven, it is often an internal force caused by our inner thoughts of imagined scenarios and unfounded fears. Regardless of whether your fears are real or imagined, the body reacts to the thought as though it was a real experience, creating a nearly unstoppable cascade of stress hormones.

Learning that your state of mind is largely dependent on what you choose to think about, is the beginning of empowering yourself to eliminate unnecessary stress during your pregnancy and for the rest of your life.

External Causes of Stress

Despite the fact that much of our stress is internal, there are triggers of stress that can arise from external events and situations, stressful psychological environments and adverse physical conditions such as pain or extreme temperatures. External stress often evaporates once the situation has been resolved or has changed.

Work

Work is often one of the leading causes of stress. High demands, long hours and long commutes can raise your stress levels until they are unmanageable.

Interpersonal work relationships can also contribute to additional stress when conflicts or disharmony arises. Pregnancy can make these typical stresses even more intense if you are feeling hormonally or physically challenged.

Relationship Issues

Divorce, marital problems, an abusive relationship, misunderstandings, poor communication and indifference from your partner can all lead to a high level of a stress during your pregnancy. In the event of a divorce or leaving an abusive relationship, use the support network around you, such as family, to ease as much stress as possible.

Unmanaged stress can also erode a relationship. It is important for each person to minimize stress to nurture a healthy relationship with the other. You can work on this together as a team, but ultimately you are each responsible for your own response and strategies to eliminate stress. If you need support as a couple, seek guidance from a counselor, relationship coach or spiritual advisor. You can even take a course in Nonviolent Communication (NVC) to improve your relationship.

Traumatic Events

Traumatic events such as a death of someone close to you, a serious illness, an accident or any negative experience that occurs suddenly and without warning can be a challenging and extremely stressful experience. If left unresolved for an extended period of time, this kind of acute stress can lead to chronic stress, which can cause damage to an individual's physical and mental health. Consequently, traumatic events and the effects of acute or chronic stress can negatively impact the health of your baby. Ensure you receive appropriate emotional counseling for any traumatic emotional or physical events. In addition, rest as much as possible and support yourself physically with healthy, whole foods such as veggies, greens and fruit.

Pregnancy

Finding out that you are pregnant can be a series of emotional highs and lows. Remember that eustress (positive stress) is often experienced when you begin to feel the excitement and joy of being pregnant.

Distress can also be felt when you find out that you are pregnant. Worries and complications during pregnancy can lead to a higher level of stress. When you compound pregnancy stress onto other sources of stress, it can lead to chronic stress, which is very harmful for both you and your baby.

Moving

Moving or selling a home can be a huge stress for most people. When you are pregnant, that stress can intensify, as the tendency during pregnancy is to nest. If it is possible, it is better not to plan any major moves during pregnancy or for at least six months after birthing, especially if a move takes you away from the support system that you have established.

Lack of a Support System

Lacking a supportive relationship, being single, living far away from family or not knowing anyone where you live can all lead to additional stress during your pregnancy. It is important to find a support group or a sense of community that can help you through your prenatal experience in a supportive way. Try to find other expecting women in prenatal classes or at local community centers that you can meet with to establish support.

Pregnancy Complications

Spotting, gestational diabetes, emergency cesarean and fetal distress can contribute to a spike of acute stress and can lead to further complications. Remember that some of these complications can be the result of too much stress in your life so trying to manage your stress levels before you get to this stage will help prevent it. However, if pregnancy complications arise, managing your stress effectively will help keep these problems from becoming worse.

Internal Causes of Stress

Internal causes of stress come from inside us and can be either physical, such as nutritional deficiencies, hormonal imbalances, illnesses, infections or inflammation. Or they can be psychological, such as worries, attitudes, beliefs, thoughts, feelings, imaginations and memories.

In addition, psychological stress can be either real or perceived. Worries over the health of the baby can be very real when you experience prenatal health complications. However, anxiety over the health of the baby when there are no complications is considered perceived and not real. Regardless, perceived stress affects you the same way as real stress.

Physical & Emotional Changes

Pregnancy comes with a number of different physical side effects that may include a range of experiences including hormonal surges, emotional outbursts, morning sickness, hair growth, cramping, an expanding belly, breast tenderness and growth, physical discomfort or changes in sex drive. Remember that most of the pregnancy related changes occurring in your body are temporary. Do the best you can to rest, eat well and to take care of your needs to prevent additional stress.

Parenting Doubts

Doubts and worries about being a parent are often a significant source of internal stress during pregnancy. Even if the pregnancy is planned, you may find yourself contemplating your ability to be able to support and effectively parent your child to be. Often expecting moms and dads may find themselves asking:

- Am I ready to be a parent?

- Is now the right time to have a baby?

- How will having a baby affect my life?

- Will I be a good mom or dad?

- Will I be able to handle the responsibilities of being a parent?

- How will a new baby affect our finances?

It is quite normal for new parents to have doubts. Your contemplation shows your concern for your child, which is a good sign. Use positive self-talk to remind yourself that, although 'fear of the unknown' has you questioning yourself, you are more than capable of raising your child. The key to being a great parent is to be a loving one. Your love will inform your decisions and guide you throughout your child's life. If you need more preparation, read books on topics such as "Attachment Parenting" or books by authors such as Dr. Dan Siegel.

Also, take the time to confide in your partner. It is a great opportunity to develop a deeper level of intimacy through expressing your vulnerability and listening to your partner's concerns and worries. If you are a single parent, share your concerns with supportive friends, family or a prenatal support group.

Pregnancy Fears

There are often many fears that arise throughout the pregnancy around the well-being of the baby. Some of the common fears expecting women experience include:

- **Will I miscarry?** Concerns about pregnancy loss are very common for expecting women, especially in the first trimester. Most miscarriages are spontaneous and unexplainable, and can result from a chromosomal abnormality, so there is little you can do to prevent them. The best thing you can do is to maintain a positive state of mind throughout your pregnancy. Worrying can create a stress response in the body, potentially contributing to a miscarriage.

- **Am I doing something that will hurt my baby?** If you are following a healthy diet, resting, exercising the right amount and avoiding alcohol, caffeine, drugs and cigarettes, then for the most part worrying is unfounded and harmful to the baby. Some common concerns include:

  o *Sex* - If you are concerned about sex affecting your baby and you are not experiencing spotting or other conditions, you can relax by knowing your baby is protected by amniotic fluid and will not be affected when you have intercourse. However, the baby may feel mild tightening when you experience an orgasm.

o *Jumping* – Vigorous or jarring movements carry some risks; so high impact sports and aerobics are not recommended. However, your general movement is not harmful to the baby.

o *Hair & nail treatments* – It is best to avoid getting hair and nail treatments in the first trimester, as the fetus is most vulnerable. I suggest avoiding these places all together throughout your pregnancy, unless they have sufficient ventilation, as the toxic chemical fumes that you inhale, from not only your treatment but also other women's treatments, can affect the development of your baby.

- **Will my baby be born healthy?** With the many prenatal tests they suggest during pregnancy, especially if you are over 35 years old, expecting moms can start to get a little focused on the status and health of their baby. If your doctor or midwife hasn't expressed concern, relax and trust in the wisdom of your body and your baby's development. Drink plenty of water, sleep as much as you feel you need to, eat a healthy balanced diet and rest frequently. In the event that a complication arises, allowing stress to overwhelm you will only aggravate a problem. Instead, stay calm, do your best to follow professional advice and take care of your needs.

- **Will embarrassing things happen during birthing?** Some women worry that embarrassing situations will arise during their birthing, such as their bowels emptying or having private areas exposed. However, the prenatal staff has seen it all before. It is just part of their work. Most women I've spoken with after their delivery have expressed the lack of concern over embarrassing issues when they are in the midst of birthing, as their energy is exclusively focused on birthing.

When pregnant for the first time, expecting moms may worry about birthing. With the combination of others experiences, advice from relatives and influence from the entertainment industry, you may have expectations based on a limited understanding of birthing. Let go of all of those influences and create a birth plan for you and your baby that is positive and nourishing. There are great books by Ina May Gaskin, and many other positive birthing advocates, that share unique and positive and pain free birthing experiences to inspire you.

It is important to discuss your birthing options with your prenatal team. You can envision a wonderful birth and stay flexible in how everything unfolds, as delivery doesn't always happen according to plans. Educate yourself about the potential complications to empower you rather than to disempower you. It will allow you to better plan for possibilities. The key is to not worry, obsess or think about things that are not real. The fantasies of negative outcomes can create those situations, as stress is the biggest contributing factor in many complications.

Additional Advice

Take each day as it comes. If you find yourself worried or anxious, look deeper to get a sense of what is at the root of the stress for you personally. Once you understand how your stress affects you personally and what triggers your stress, then you can use this book to journey through your own stress and find the peace and enjoyment that pregnancy brings.

Before you embark on the journey, however, I recommend that you sit down and write five things you deal with on a daily basis that frustrate you or leave you feeling overwhelmed and full of tension. Once you have those five things written down, decide if you can cut back on your exposure. Can you opt out of anything? Is there someone who can assist you and share in your responsibility? Can you take a medical leave from work? Think about how you can make positive and nourishing changes in your pregnancy.

Next, write a new list of five things that help you relax. Make sure that they are all healthy for both you and your baby. Activities such as taking a soothing, warm bath or going for a nice walk around the neighborhood are good choices. Let the strategies in this book be a resource to assist you to explore ways to help you to eliminate stress, relax and experience well-being and peace throughout your prenatal journey.

Note: The strategies in this book are great tools to resolve stressors. Use them to transform your stressed states into empowered experiences. If you are experiencing chronic stress or severe symptoms of stress, consult with your health care professional immediately.

108 Tips for Enjoying Your Prenatal Journey

It's not what you go through that defines you; you can't help that.
It's what you do AFTER you've gone through it that really
tests who you are.

~*Kwame Floyd*

Congratulations! Not only are you expecting a baby, but you are also taking empowering steps to make your pregnancy as wonderful as it can be. As with life in general, situations and events can pop up during your pregnancy that may feel challenging and stressful.

Use the suggestions and strategies throughout this book to assist you to eliminate, manage, prevent and transform any stress that arises, so you can simply enjoy your pregnancy in a peaceful way. Enjoy!

Believe in You

Birth is an opportunity to transcend. To rise above what we are accustomed to, reach deeper inside ourselves than we are familiar with, and to see not only what we are truly made of, but the strength we can access in and through birth.

~ Marcie Macari

You are an amazing being. Among all your gifts, you've been given the gift to experience the extraordinary blessing of nurturing and birthing a new soul into existence.

If you are feeling fearful and worried about your abilities as a new mom, you are not alone. Many new expecting moms experience self-doubt because pregnancy is a totally new experience that takes a woman out of what is known and comfortable. Even women who experience multiple pregnancies experience some doubt and anxiety with each pregnancy because no two pregnancies are the same.

Unfortunately, negative self-talk creates stress for both you and your baby. However, you have the opportunity transform negative self-talk to positive self-talk. The key is to consciously cultivate and strengthen your belief in your abilities in your new role as a mom.

First, change your mind! Take a stand that you will believe in yourself regardless of what you've thought in the past or what thoughts may pop up throughout your pregnancy.

Second, right now, allow yourself to say out loud, *"I am a beautiful, intelligent, strong and capable woman. I choose to shine my light throughout my pregnancy and after my baby is born. What I don't know, I will find the appropriate resources and*

educate myself. As I learn and grow, I implement new wisdom to do the very best I can for
myself and my baby."

Third, if you find it difficult to really focus on the positive aspects that make you uniquely you, take the time to write them down and affirm them every day. Place them on sticky notes and put them in a place where you will see them.

Fourth, explore this book to empower you throughout your pregnancy. I have included over a hundred tips to assist you to give you tools to believe in yourself to transform your prenatal journey into one that is peaceful and meaningful.

Fifth, let go of any ideas of 'perfection' and give up the myth of other peoples' ideas of the 'ideal' pregnancy. The ideal choices align with what is best for your baby. In all your decision making ask, "What would be the best decision for my baby at this time?" or "What is the healthiest choice for my baby at this time?" This begins your role as 'mom,' as most mothers consider what is best for their children when they approach a situation.

Believing in yourself and your future is the first step in how you move through your pregnancy stress free. By believing in yourself, that confidence translates into a more peaceful experience for you and your baby. You are an amazing person and you have the ability in be an amazing mother starting from today regardless of your past experiences or lack of experience as a mom. Now is the time to really believe in you!

Remember Billions of Women
Have Done This Before

Women…are storytellers. They are nurturers…filled with creative forces when they are fertile, pregnant or birthing. Millions of years of biology are on their side to 'bring forth.' Nothing can stop the power behind that force, not even the woman herself… She is the living essence of the future. She is a holy woman and there is intelligence at work in her. It is sacred energy.

~ Sister MorningStar

In known history, over 108 billion human births have occurred. There are over 21 million births per year. There are more than 300,000 births per day. There are more than 4.17 births per second. As you give birth to your child, at least three other babies are being born at the same time.

Birth is an ancient celebration. Every aspect of a women's being is encoded with the natural process of childbirth. You are connected to an ancient lineage of women who have given birth. Allow yourself to feel into this powerful bond to the energy of *sacred mother*.

Celebrate Your Pregnancy

The more you praise and celebrate your life, the more there is in life to celebrate.

~ Oprah Winfrey

Your prenatal journey can be a wonderful time to celebrate. Cherish your role as the powerful nourisher and protector of the little baby within you. Celebrate your role as a co-creator with all of existence. Creation is enfolding within you every moment of your pregnancy. A new soul has chosen you to be its mom. You and your baby's life are intertwined in a nine-month dance that will change you for the rest of your life.

Pregnancy is a unique event that most women experience only one to three times in their lifetime. The opportunity to enjoy being pregnant with the baby within you only happens once. After giving birth, I have heard many women express that they would have liked to have been more patient while pregnant and taken the time to be more present to enjoy the sensations and changes they were experiencing. Revere the moments that you spend together and take time to simply celebrate each prenatal experience along the way.

You may have ups and downs during your pregnancy as hormones fluctuate and your body changes. Learn to find a place of acceptance for days that may be more challenging than others. Acceptance is celebrating 'what is,' rather than being in a state of wanting things to be different.

A simple exercise of celebration to inspire you during your pregnancy:

Life is worth rejoicing every day. When you wake each morning and go to bed at night, celebrate the blessing of your baby within you by raising your arms up above your head in a 'Y' shape. Then say, "Thank you, thank you, thank you." Your body is in a position of receptivity, forming a chalice like shape, which informs the universe that you are open to receive its blessings. This exercise can also be done anytime, but is especially powerful when done in nature.

Take Baby Steps

It is better to take many small steps in the right direction than to make
a great leap forward only to stumble backward.

~*Old Chinese Proverb*

Every journey begins with a step. Your prenatal journey begins with education. Set aside time to educate yourself so you will have an idea of how you'd like to experience your pregnancy and the birth of your baby. Read prenatal books, watch positive birthing videos and learn from women with affirming birth experiences to get a larger perspective about pregnancy and birthing.

When you've had a chance to learn more about you and your baby's needs during the different stages of pregnancy, begin to brainstorm your blueprint for a peaceful and nourishing pregnancy that involves strategies for nutrition, stress reduction, rest, relaxation, work and exercise.

After you have learned about the various options for birthing your baby, sketch out your birthing plan to reflect the type of birth you believe would be ideal. Remember to also have a contingency plan available in case events unfold differently. See section "Develop a Birthing Plan" for more details.

Implement your pregnancy strategies and birthing plan as your pregnancy progresses, while staying flexible to experiences and events that you may not have considered. Plans can always be adjusted as new information or issues arise.

Do the best you can do in any given moment. Let go of the need to figure everything out right now or to do things perfectly. Worrying about any stage of your pregnancy or the birthing process can create a cycle of stress that is harmful to your baby, sometimes creating the very thing you want to avoid. Instead, build on and celebrate all of your successes, even the small ones.

You can use the strategy of taking baby steps in all areas of your life. Implement projects a little at a time. Take breaks in between each step to refresh yourself with any of the strategies you learn in this book and then carry on with the project. If you can't get something done by the end of the day, don't worry about it. The reality in life is that there will always be something more to do, but you can choose today to take it in healthy, measured steps.

Educate > Plan > Implement > Let Go

Breathe

I am open to receive with every breath I breathe.

~ Michael Sun

Breathing is essential to life. In times of stress, the tendency is for people to hold their breath, which creates a state of contraction and limits the amount of oxygen that gets to the cells of the brain and body. Shallow, constricted breathing is an unhealthy pattern of breathing just to survive. Deep, full breathing allows the body to thrive. When you are pregnant, you are breathing for both you and your baby, so it is essential to establish healthy breathing patterns.

The first step to healthy breathing is awareness. From time to time, observe how you are breathing, especially if you are feeling stressed. Does the breath move easily into your belly and your lungs? Are you breathing deeply and slowly? If not, take a moment, breathe in slowly, pause and then slowly let it go. Watch your breath as it moves in and out of your body. How does it feel?

Healthy, natural breathing helps with circulation by opening capillaries to allow blood to flow through the body. It assists the mind and body to enter into a state of relaxation and can help reverse the effects of stress. A deep breath today can undo the effects worrying and has been linked to alleviating the side effects of:

- Heart Disease
- Inability to Concentrate
- Tension
- Headache
- Fatigue
- Anxiety
- Depression
- Sleeping Problems

Learning how to focus your breathing helps to alleviate stress during your pregnancy and gives you strategies for managing pain during the birthing process. Take a Lamaze course, Hypnobirthing class or a birthing class to learn helpful breathing techniques for childbirth to help with pain management and to assist you to breathe your baby out. Conscious breathing is also a great tool to help you manage your stress when you are a new parent. Apply the following breathing techniques any time you feel stressed.

The Sitting Breath

The Sitting Breath is an excellent breathing method that can be used just about anywhere – in the car, at a park, on the bus, in the office or at home. The benefit of the Sitting Breath exercise is that it directs the breath to go down your entire body to relieve the tension that results from stress.

1. Place yourself in a comfortable sitting position. Make sure that your back is straight.

2. If you can close your eyes, do so. If you don't feel comfortable closing your eyes, look at something in the distance; this will be your focal point.

3. Take a deep breath in. The proper way to do this is to relax the muscles of your abdomen and allow your belly to fill with air. If you place your hands on your abdomen, your stomach should expand with the breath.

4. Hold the breath to the slow count of five, but exhale it before if starts to cause you discomfort.

5. Exhale slowly. Your abdomen should contract as you exhale and you should be able to relax your chest. Breathe out from your belly. When you are learning this exercise, it is better to place your hand over your belly as you breathe out to remind yourself to breathe from that point.

6. Allow your body to relax as you exhale the breath and try to focus on just the breathing as it goes in and out slowly. Relax your mind and only think of the cleansing breath.

7. Continue this for five minutes or until you feel your body relax.

Breath Counting

Another easy and effective breathing exercise that you can do anywhere is Breath Counting. This method of relaxation works to distract the mind by having you focus on something else. It can be done sitting, standing or lying down.

1. Find a position that is comfortable for you.

2. Inhale slowly and hold it for a moment and exhale slowly. Count... "One."

3. Inhale slowly, hold it for a moment and exhale slowly. Count... "Two."

4. Inhale again, hold it and exhale slowly. Count... "Three."

5. Repeat this until you get to ten. Count each exhale and not the inhale. Once you have reached ten, start again at one.

6. Continue for 5 to 10 minutes.

Connect With Your Higher Power

As your faith is strengthened you will find that there is no longer the need to have a sense of control, that things will flow as they will, and that you will flow with them, to your great delight and benefit.

~Emmanuel Teney

When I reflect on my life, nature and the universe, I begin to realize that there is such an intricate wisdom that is unfathomable. From the miracle of life and the mysteries of energy to the interconnectedness of all of creation, I rejoice in gratitude for the experiences that I have enjoyed so far. When we are young, we think we know it all. Yet we know next to nothing about how and why things are as they are. I delight in nature's secrets being revealed. And I love when I notice something new and become reborn with the wonder of a child. It is a profound reminder that the Creator of all things is a creative and artistic architect.

Depending on your culture and the language you speak, there are thousands of different names for the Creator: Ahura Mazda, Almighty, Allah, Brahman, Creator, the Divine, Ehyeh, Ek Onkar, El, Elaha, Great Spirit, God, the Highest God, I AM, Iesus, Indra, Ishvar, Jesus, Krishna, The Light, Lord, Rama, Shen, Tian Zhu, Vishnu, Waheguru, Yahweh, Yeshua, YHWH and many more.

Regardless of anyone else's relationship with the Creator, your relationship is unique to you. Whether or not you believe in a higher creative force, be aware that we are connected with everyone and everything in this universe.

For those who believe in a loving Creator, the relationship can be a comforting one especially in times of stress and uncertainty. Having a personal relationship with the Creator is a powerful way to overcome the stress and worry about your unborn child by sharing your concerns and giving over your worries. If you are up at night with a million thoughts keeping you up, just connect with the Creator and envision yourself handing over your negative thoughts to be handled for you. If more come up, give those over, too.

Many people express that peace is often achieved through communion with their faith. There are many ways to connect with the Creator: prayer, being in nature, meditation, reflection, dancing, singing, compassion, love and many other creative expressions.

Live life in celebration and extend the love that you feel through your faith to those around you and to your unborn child. Be grateful for all that you have and everything that has been provided for you.

Connect With the Wisdom of Your Soul

When enough women realize that birth is a time of great opportunity to get in touch with their true power, and when they are willing to assume responsibility for this, we will reclaim the power of birth and help move technology where it belongs— in the service of birthing women, not their master.

~ *Christiane Northrup*

Most people have a sense of self, but not a full realization of who they are as a Soul. Some people think that they are their body or brain and when they die they cease to exist. However, billions of people have an intuitive sense that there is more to who they are beyond the body and brain.

Some blessed ones have caught a glimpse of their Soul. Then there are the enlightened and holy people who have experienced Self-realization and even God-realization and true knowledge of the Soul.

There are many names in many languages for the higher self: Aatma, Atman, Buddha nature, Chetena, Essence, Eternal Soul, I AM, Jeev, Jiva, Pure Self, Ruh, Soul, Spirit, Tao, True Self and Timeless Self. Regardless of the names, most traditions in the world reflect on the existence and importance of the Soul, as well as regarding it as our true state and true self.

41

In the Hindu tradition, sacred texts reveal that the true soul is considered eternal and incorruptible. "It [the immutable soul] is not born, It does not die, at no time did It come into being, nor will It come into being hereafter. It is unborn, eternal, permanent and ancient. It is not killed when the body is slain…This soul cannot be severed by weapons, burnt by fire, wetted with water, nor dried by the wind. It is unbreakable, unburnable, It cannot be wetted nor dried. It is eternal and all-pervading, equable, immovable and eternally constant." (Bhagavad Gita 2:20, 23, 24)

According to many traditions, including Sikhism, the soul is considered to be a part of God. "The soul is divine; divine is the soul. Worship Him with love."[11] Also, "The soul is the Lord, and the Lord is the soul; contemplating the Shabad, the Lord is found."[12]

Christian passages also reveal the connection of the soul to God, "And the dust returns to the earth as it was, and the spirit returns to God who gave it." (Ecclesiastes 12:7) Jesus also shares the profound importance of the soul in relationship to God as we live this life: "You shall love the Lord your God with all your heart and with all your soul and with all your strength and with all your mind, and your neighbor as yourself." (Luke 10:27) And, in a letter to the Galatians, the New Testament of the Bible itemizes the fruits of the Spirit as: love, joy, peace, patience, kindness, generosity, faithfulness, gentleness and self-control.

Although some would suggest that Buddhism denies the existence of a soul through the concept of anatta or 'no self', the teachings really share the profound concept of a non-material soul and steers people away from the idea of the soul being 'something.' The Buddhist concept of 'consciousness' that is free of any idea of permanence or selfhood would describe what others might consider the soul. I suspect that what is being presented is a viewpoint to assist the human mind to let go of any illusionary concepts it has about existence. Anyway, the more I write about this, the more I realize that describing the soul is a vain attempt to describe the indescribable.

Just like there is an umbilical cord connecting an unborn baby to its mother, it is believed in many spiritual traditions that there is an energetic cord that connects our physical body to our Soul.

When you are connected with your Higher Self or Soul:
- You reside in a peaceful state because you are free of agitation, happiness, excitedness, stress, distraction and disturbances.
- You are in the present moment state of feeling connected.
- You reside in a state of clarity because little influences you.
- You feel guided.
- You experience gratitude.
- You are aware that everything has been a gift and has brought you to this moment.

When you are disconnected from your Higher Self:
- You are in the mind's ideas of rightness and wrongness.
- You are attached to expectations and ideas of how things should be.
- You experience dissatisfaction, disappointment and frustration.
- You feel anxious and stressed.
- You experience confusion, agitation, frustration, anger and rage.
- You are influenced by people, social and cultural conditioning, past experiences, ideas of the future and learned beliefs.
- You are influenced by fear and ideas of not being good enough.

Ways to connect with your Higher Self:

- Connect to the heart by focusing your breath and attention on the heart center.

- Pray and ask for Divine guidance.

- Practice asking questions and listening for answers, which most likely will come as a soft, peaceful inner voice or could appear as a sign throughout your day.

- Find fellowship with those who are aligned with their Higher Self.

- Read sacred texts.

- Recite mantras, spiritual songs or prayers – A mantra can be a syllable, a sound, a word, or words that are repeated to create transformation. Mantras can be spoken, whispered, hummed, and sung out loud or quietly within the mind. There are many traditions of reciting mantras from around the world such as:

- **Lord's Prayer** - Our Father in heaven, hallowed be your name. Your kingdom come, your will be done, on earth as it is in heaven. Give us this day our daily bread and forgive us our trespasses, as we forgive those who trespass against us. And lead us not into temptation, but deliver us from evil. Amen.

- **Marantha** - MA-RA-NA-THA is Aramaic for "Come Lord" (from the *New Testament Book of Revelations*).

- **God's Light** - God's Light, God's Light, God's Light, God's Light, …

- **Islamic Kalma** - LA ILAHA IL LAL LAHU MUHAMMADUR RASULULLAH, which translates to "None but the One true God is worthy of worship. Muhammad is His Messenger."

- **Om or Aum** - ॐ - "I am existence," the name of God, the word of God, the vibration of the Supreme, the first and original vibration or "word of God" manifesting as the sound "OM."
- **Om Mani Padme Hum** - refers to the "Jewel in the Lotus." This mantra represents achieving the perfection of generosity, pure ethics, tolerance, patience, perseverance, concentration and wisdom.

Listen To the Wisdom of Your Body

Our body-wisdom knows how to birth a baby. What is required of the woman who births naturally is for her to surrender to this body-wisdom. You can't think your way through a birth, and you can't fake it.

~ Leslie McIntyre

Your body and brain are perfectly designed to operate without any direction from you. Each cell of the body has its function and is equipped to fulfill the blueprint it has been given, unless you throw a monkey wrench into the mix through excess stress, poor nutrition, overexertion or exposure to environmental toxins.

Listening to the wisdom of your body and mind is about bringing your awareness to the ways they speak to you and finding strategies and practices that bring balance into your life. Communication can reveal itself as a nagging idea, a physical sensation, a discomfort, a mood, a state of mind, exhaustion or even a symptom of disease. During pregnancy, bringing awareness to the body's wisdom is practice for getting in touch with body-wisdom when birthing your baby.

Not heeding forewarnings from your body and mind is a recipe for major health issues and prenatal complications for you and your baby. The good news is that these warning signs assist you to pin point where your attention is best needed to resolve the issue effectively. As soon as you are aware of the symptoms of stress in the body or mind, it is important to address their root cause. By learning to listen, you become more attuned to what your body asks for moment to moment.

A great way to listen to your body and mind is to sit down somewhere quiet to relax. Gently breathe in and out of your nose, filling your abdomen while maintaining awareness of your breath. If you feel any areas of constriction, tightness or soreness, gently breathe into those areas. As you feel yourself relax, ask: "What do I need to do in this moment to take care of my body and mind?" The answer will come to you...all you have to do is listen.

Honor Your Emotions

Emotion is the chief source of becoming-conscious. There can be no transforming of darkness into light and of apathy into movement without emotion.

~ Carl Jung

Strong emotions like fear, anger and sadness are normal reactions to the human experience. However, we are erroneously taught to hide our emotions, to deny ourselves the expression of them or to express them in destructive ways. Often these harmful repression patterns are ancestrally and culturally passed on from generation to generation. Unresolved emotional conflicts and traumas are the root of most emotional issues, stress, physical injuries and disease.

When you push your emotions down or away, rather than releasing them from you, they become anchored in you. To prevent further repression of your emotions, begin to feel what you are experiencing and find acceptance without self-judgment. You can ask yourself some investigative questions: Why might I be feeling angry? What is at the root of this sadness? What fear might this situation be triggering in me? Which of my needs is not being met at this time?

To heal and release repressed emotions use strategies such as:

- Emotional Freedom Technique to release current or past trapped emotions.
- Journaling and writing to express yourself.
- Art therapy to creatively express yourself.
- Crying to release pain, hurt and stress. As you cry, be sure to say to your self, "I am feeling _____."
- Joining a support group or receiving some counseling to give voice to your emotions.
- **Suggested reading -** *Codependent No More* by Melody Beattie

Identify Your Stressors

Stress is inner biofeedback, signaling you that frequencies are fighting within your system.
The purpose of stress isn't to hurt you, but to let you know it's
time to go back to the heart and start loving.

~ *Sara Paddison*

Do you ever reflect at the end of your day on how busy you were but felt like you accomplished very little? Have you ever felt so exhausted by all you had to do and feel as though you are getting nowhere? Are there people in your life that seem to zap your energy? Where has all your time and energy gone today?

People, work, situations and experiences can trigger a stress response in your body. Stressors can come from anywhere and one of the most common places is from within. Depending on how you set up your life, you may be feeling overwhelmed, exhausted and even stressed by all the thoughts running around inside your head or by the activities you've chosen to participate in.

There are activities that seem to nourish you and then there are those that seem to sap the strength from you. Worry over your relationships and how your baby is growing are often at the top of the list of reasons why expecting moms feel stressed. However, sometimes those worries are not the root of the problem, so it is important to identify the root causes of your anxiety and stress so you can manage or eliminate the stress. Ask yourself:

1. **What activities, thoughts or situations drain you?** People are not always aware of where their energy is going, so it is important to identify your stressors to shine the light of awareness upon the

48

situation. Sit down and jot down the different issues and stresses in your life. Don't be afraid to list everything, no matter how small they may seem. Organize the list into minor and major issues. Eventually, you will have a refined list that will help you identify what is causing most of your stress. Once you have identified your stressors, begin to find solutions or eliminate the root causes. Use Emotional Freedom Technique (review the section called "Use Emotional Freedom Technique") to release stuck emotional energy related to these stressors.

2. **What am I avoiding or neglecting?** You may be avoiding completing a task or neglecting to resolve a conflict or even put off taking some time for relaxation. When you avoid issues, their presence still works as an energy drain, pulling our attention until the situation is resolved or completed. By taking the time to complete any minor or major tasks you have been putting off, you'll experience an increase in energy and a sense of freedom.

3. **What aspects of my life do I enjoy?** Now that you have a list of things that are causing you stress, make a list of the activities that you love to do and that nourish you the most. While you still need to correct the draining energies, it is good to identify the things that will recharge your energy when you feel drained. Take the time each day to do something nourishing.

Draining energies can be:

- **Internal -** Negative thoughts and emotions are a major source of stress. If your issue is compulsive worrying, get some help from a professional who is trained at eliminating compulsive behaviors. I also offer some helpful strategies throughout this book for transforming negative thoughts into positive ones.

- **Environmental -** Clutter, an unclean house, disruptive people, background and television noise or not having a quiet place in your home can be draining. Your home is a sanctuary. Create a peaceful environment by keeping your spaces free of clutter, fixing anything that is broken and turning the TV off unless you are tuning in to a specific program. Invite only those who provide a positive energy into your home.

- **Idle activities -** Chitchat, texting, playing games, Internet surfing, social media and email can waste large amounts of time when pooled together over a day. Turn off your ringer, stop unnecessary texting and check your emails a few times per day. Let go of the need to be perpetually available to everyone. Set time limits for these activities. You may find yourself more relaxed and better focused with your day.

- **Work -** The workplace can be a big drain on energy if you don't balance work with fun and rest. Make sure you take breaks regularly and go outside to get a little sunshine and some fresh air. Enjoy fun activities after work such as yoga or going for a walk with a friend. It is important to identify ways to eliminate unnecessary stress. This could be anything from cleaning up your desk to addressing a workplace bully issue or even letting go of any need to change a co-worker's behavior. If you feel stressed because of an unresolved issue at work, find a peaceful way to resolve the situation. If you find conflict resolution difficult, ask for help from a colleague or mentor.

If work stress is affecting your health, talk to your doctor about a medical leave of absence.

- **Relationships** - How we connect with the people in our lives can be draining, so it is important to figure out how you can make your relationships healthier. Address any unresolved issues and, if they cannot be fixed, find a way to co-exist or move on from any unhealthy relationships. The biggest key is to let others be free of your judgment and influence and choose to be free of their judgment and influence. If you do that, you'll be surprised at how peaceful life can be when co-existing together. If there are people in your life who are negative or hurtful, it is better to not spend time with them during your pregnancy, if possible.

- **Health** - Unhealthy food, health issues, trying to control things, not sleeping and constant worrying will drain your energy quickly. Find solutions and healthy ways to establish balance in your body and mind.

- **Commitments** - Cut out any unnecessary commitments you have chosen to busy yourself with. Find ways to politely and confidently say 'no' if someone asks you to volunteer or join an activity. Choose activities that leave you with more energy. Free up time to rest and get important tasks completed. Schedule blocks of time for yourself in your calendar to ensure you don't book unnecessary activities. You can then tell people you have something planned for that time slot...your sanity!

- **Pregnancy** - Pregnancy itself brings about a number of physical, emotional and energetic stressors. As internal resources are being used for the development of your baby, accept that you may experience limits to your normal abilities. Resting and meeting your basic needs gives you the necessary resources for you and your baby. Be realistic about what you can achieve and can commit to doing during your day.

Use Emotional Freedom Technique

The cause of all negative emotions is a disruption in the body's energy system.

~ Gary Craig, Founder of EFT

I highly recommend Emotional Freedom Technique (EFT), as it has been one of the most effective strategies I have personally come across. EFT is easy to learn and use for a variety of traumas, emotional experiences and stressful situations.

EFT is a simple method of lightly tapping on traditional acupressure points on the body without needles. The light tapping on specific points on the head and chest combined with verbal phrases specific to your issue works to clear the emotional conflict from your body's energy system. In most cases, EFT helps to restore the mind-body balance creating an optimum state for healing.

Research studies have revealed significant reductions in anxiety,[13] stress, depression, post-traumatic stress,[14] and traumatic memories when people use EFT. In addition, researchers have observed the neurochemical benefits of the stimulation of acupressure points that include the regulation of the stress hormone called cortisol, as well as the increase of production of endorphins, serotonin and gamma-aminobutyric acid (GABA).[15] [16] [17] These neurochemical changes cause a cascade of relaxation and a reduction of pain and anxiety. They slow the heart rate, shut off the fear induced flight-fight-freeze response and create a sense of calm.[18] [19]

For minor stress relief, you can administer EFT on your own. If you have acute or chronic stress, anxiety or unresolved emotional conflicts, I recommend that you work with a qualified EFT practitioner. Many counselors, psychologists and therapists are incorporating EFT into their work due to its effectiveness. Depending on where you live there are most likely many people available to assist you. EFT practitioners work online as well.

Basic EFT

The three basic elements you need to learn for the purpose of using EFT are:
- Which acupressure points to tap.
- How to tap the points.
- The phrases to say while tapping.

It is easier to learn EFT by video demonstration. If you'd like an online demo, visit www.stress-free-pregnancy.com/eft. If you have unresolved emotional conflicts and stress around pregnancy, visit www.stress-free-pregnancy.com /courses for details on prenatal coaching or the **EFT for Baby & Me** online course.

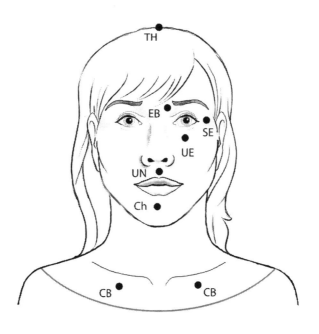

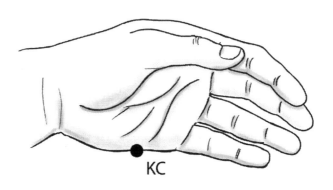

The specific points that you will tap are:

- The soft spot on the side of your hand, known as the Karate Chop (KC) point, located half way between your wrist bone and the bone below your pinky

- On top of the head (TH)

- Inner eyebrow on the bone that is just above the inner corner of the eye (EB)

- On the bone that is located on the edge of the far outside part of eye, below the end of the eyebrow (SE)

- On the bone under the center of the eye (UE)

- Under the nose but above the top lip (UN)

- In between the bottom lip and the chin (Ch)

- Just below the collarbone to the left or right of the U shaped bone below your throat (CB)

- About six inches below your armpit at the side of your body (UA)

EFT incorporates a specific formula for successfully eliminating the emotional charge around a given stress. To use EFT effectively, use these steps:

1. Identify a significant area of stress. If you are currently reacting to a stressor, focus on the experience at hand. If you can't think of one, return to the section "Identify Your Stressors" to identify the situations that are causing you the most stress at this time.

2. Use the EFT set up phrase with your stressor, "Even though
_____, I fully and completely love and accept myself." This
phrase addresses the current state of the situation, while it allows for
you to love yourself even if you are feeling emotional about an issue.
The benefit is that you accept 'what is' rather than being in a state of
wanting it to be different, which allows for that aspect of you that
feels an emotion to be heard. For example, if you are feeling angry
that your partner couldn't make it to a prenatal appointment, you
could say, *"Even though I feel angry that Bob didn't make it to our
appointment, I fully and completely love and accept myself."* Or if you felt
overwhelmed at work, you might say, *"Even though I felt overwhelmed at
work, I fully and completely love and accept myself."*

3. Once you have a phrase, you can begin tapping. Start with the Karate
Chop point on your hand and repeat the phrase three times as you
tap that point. Use light tapping to ensure you don't bruise the soft
tissue.

4. Create reminder phrases once you are done tapping at the Karate
Chop point. The reminder phrase is an abbreviated version of your
set up phrase or a related statement about your experience, however
it does not include the last part of the set up phrase. From my
example it would be something like, *"I feel angry that Bob didn't make it
to our appointment."* Additional phrases to use could include:

    a. I feel frustrated that he didn't make more of an effort.

    b. I feel annoyed that this isn't the first time.

    c. I just wanted him to be there.

    d. I just want to feel supported.

5. Repeat the tapping on each of the remaining pressure points listed in the diagram above. Change the reminder phrase to describe all your feelings, experiences and needs around the incident.

6. You can do more than one round if you have an extensive list of feelings and needs around the incident. Once you feel you've expressed them all, look at the stressor again. If it is still high, repeat the exercise until you find that your stress level is lowered significantly or eliminated.

Use Non-Violent Communication

What others do may be a stimulus of our feelings, but not the cause.

~ Marshall B. Rosenberg, Ph.D.,
Founder of NVC

I grew up in a family that didn't have healthy communication skills and my parents had a policy of 'no fighting' amongst the kids. My dad often separated us and sternly warned us that he didn't want to hear another word about whatever we were fighting over. In relationship to our parents, we were not allowed to express our needs, as it was considered talking back and there were serious consequences. We soon learned to find negative ways to cope with the emotional swamp that was brewing within us. With no healthy communication tools, the lack of the expression of our needs fostered a great deal of internalized aggression, stress and depression among our family.

Our parents did not have healthy communication skills and were unable to teach us and assist us in expressing our needs. Since our parents modeled communication by yelling to express emotions and communicate needs, my sister and I resorted to screaming and physical fighting whenever our parents were not around. It wasn't an effective tool for getting ones needs met. However, it worked at the time to release the pent up stress we felt by suppressing our emotions.

Most people have been educated from birth to repress emotions, compete, judge, demand and diagnose when communicating with others. Rather than expressing their needs in non-demanding ways, many people resort to behaviors based in terms of what another has "done to me." From this viewpoint, our relationships become tainted and our communication is ineffective. However, there are non-violent communication skills that can be learned that can change your closest relationships and can alter the way you communicate in the workplace or with people in general.

Compassionate communication is a legacy; it is a beautiful gift that can be passed on from generation to generation once it is learned. Children learn from whatever you model. Your partner will often mirror what you infuse into the relationship. If your parents modeled unhealthy forms of communication, give yourself the gift of learning non-violent communication (NVC).

NVC is a learned process, first developed by Dr. Marshall Rosenberg in the 1960s. I have provided some brief information on NVC below. However, I recommend that you take an NVC course or learn at your own pace by reading *Non-Violent Communication: A Language of Life* by Marshall B. Rosenberg Ph.D. for a more detailed understanding.

What is Non-Violent Communication?

- Learning to observe others rather than to judge or evaluate them.

- Learning to distinguish between ideas and feelings.

- Learning to identify your unmet needs as well as others unmet needs.

- Learning how to express your needs rather than focusing on what you don't want.

- Learning not to manipulate others through fear, guilt, shame or obligation.

- Learning how to listen.

- Learning to resolve conflicts with ease.

Four Components of Non-Violent Communication

The basic components of NVC are:

- Observe behavior
- Indentify feelings
- Identify needs
- Make a request

Basic Examples of the NVC Process

Here is an example of expressing how to use "I" statements without blaming or criticizing the other person:

When I see/hear you _____, I feel _____, because I need/value _____. Would you be willing to _____?

When I see you leave dirty dishes, I feel frustrated, because I need to not have to ask you to clean up after yourself. Would you be willing to rinse your dishes and put them in the dishwasher when you are done eating?

When I hear you complain about my friends, I feel sad, because I need to have time with other people. Would you be willing to express how you are feeling about me going out in non-violent ways? Would you be willing to share with me what needs of yours are not being met?

Here is an example of empathically receiving how another is without hearing blame or criticism:

When you see/hear me _____, you feel _____, because you need/value _____. Would you like _____?

When you see me not taking care of myself, you feel scared because you need me to look after my health. Would you like me to work fewer hours while I'm pregnant?

Benefits of Non-Violent Communication

The benefits of learning healthy communication tools for the expression of needs and emotions include:

- Less stress
- Improved relationships
- Healthy expression of emotions
- A sense of empowerment
- Building trust
- Healing pain
- Creating peace

Let Go of Guilt and Shame

Shame can be a powerful force in our life.
It is the trademark of dysfunctional families.

~ Melody Beattie, Language of Letting Go

Far too many people carry around guilt and shame in their lives. The stress of guilt and shame contribute to mental and physical issues and can destroy someone's life.

Guilt and shame can come from beliefs you've accepted from your parents, family, school, religion, media, advertising and society. Regardless of how repressed a person's shame may be, shame easily transfers to the next generation. Children first take on their parent's shame energetically at birth and then through learned behavior throughout childhood and adolescence.

Generational shame can be transferred without us knowing it. For example, when I was eight years old, I took on my mother's shame around being a woman. My mom was menstruating on a day that her friend came over for a cup of tea. Our unruly dog pulled out her used menstrual pads from the bathroom garbage and started to tear them up in the hallway. My mom was deeply embarrassed. I felt sorry for her, but I also took on a great deal of shame. I became aware of this shame in my mid 30s. I was glad to become aware of it so I could clear the shame to be free of it and to prevent passing it on to my children.

Although menstruation is a natural reproductive process, there is a cultural attitude that menstruation is dirty and some thing to keep secret. Many women and girls report stories where they felt incredible shame for

61

bleeding through their clothes, smelling different or being seen with menstrual products.

Shame and guilt can come from a variety of experiences throughout life. Many people use shame and guilt interchangeably, but they are not the same kind of experience. The difference between guilt and shame can be summed up with these statement comparisons:

Guilt is the acknowledgement that "I've made a mistake."

Shame is the belief that "I am a mistake."

In the case of shame, the person takes on the shame as an internalized identity. Some additional examples include: "I am worthless," "I'm a bitch," I'm evil," "I'm a failure," "Women are evil" or "I'm not good enough."

Shame can become debilitating because it creates a war within the person as they temporarily accept the shame identity at the conscious mind. The stress of carrying shame can become so unbearable that a psychological and spiritual split can occur. At that point the shame is experienced at the subconscious mind as a repressed and unconscious belief about oneself.

The imprint of shame at the unconscious level creates a false self to hide within. People with repressed shame will have tendencies to prove they are anything but the internalized shame.

So no matter what they accomplish or who they are, their repressed shame will create one or more of the following conditions: alienation, compulsive disorders, depression, inadequacy, inferiority, isolating loneliness, self doubt, sense of failure, superiority, paranoia, perfectionism and more.

Steps to Begin Healing Shame

1. The first step in healing shame is to learn to identify it. Do you catch yourself making statements such as "**I am** no good" or "**I'm** a failure"?

62

2. Realize that you have personally identified with an idea about yourself and then change your idea to "**I believe** I am no good."

3. Clear the statements using EFT (review the section called "Use Emotional Freedom Technique"). While tapping say, "Even though **I believe I am no good,** I fully and completely love and accept myself." Or "Even though I _____, I fully and completely love and accept myself."

4. Give yourself and others permission to make mistakes.

5. Connect with a higher power, ask for forgiveness and let your higher power take care of the forgiveness.

6. Take a stand and choose to love yourself and use positive self-talk to begin cultivating happiness.

7. Get present and get real. What are the facts of the present moment without judgment or entertaining negative stories about you from the past?

8. Get support. If you experience shame, find a support group or a counseling practitioner who can assist you to release your shame.

9. Read more about shame. I highly recommend John Bradshaw's book, *Healing the Shame that Binds You.* He does a great job in describing shame and suggests many tools to heal shame.

Ways to Transform Guilt

It is time to let go of any guilt you are carrying. Guilt is highly stressful, energetically expensive and totally unnecessary once we know how to transform it. Maya Angelou summed it up best when she said, "You did what you knew how to do, and when you knew better, you did better."

We have all done things for which we judge ourselves. Feeling guilty doesn't make things better, so take responsibility and take steps to clear the guilt. Here are the steps to transform guilt:

1. **Identify the Guilt** – If you're ready, let's begin. Write down what are you feeling guilty about. Realize that guilt is an indication that there is something unresolved in your mind.

2. **Take Responsibility** – Have you been hurtful to your self or others? Are you feeling guilty for not following through with something you wanted to do or said you would do? Are you ready to do something about the guilt?

3. **Make Amends** – If you've done something to harm someone, then make amends in the most appropriate way. This could be to apologize or make up for your actions. If the person is no longer in your life or has passed away, you can make amends by doing something in their honor like planting a tree or giving to charity. You can also ask for forgiveness by using the Ho'oponopono Prayer of Forgiveness (see section "Practice Forgiveness). In addition to making amends, the most important step is to correct your behavior if you are continuously acting in hurtful ways to yourself or others.

4. **Acceptance** – If you've done something hurtful and you have made amends, then move on. Accept that you cannot change the past and let go of the need to feel guilty. Forgive yourself and others.

5. **Learning** – When we allow ourselves to learn from past mistakes, we have the ability to make new choices in the future. Past mistakes are indicators to assist us in self-correcting to ensure we are on the path that we want to be on. You may even experience gratitude in your learning opportunities.

6. **Review** – See some of the suggestions in the section above on **Steps to Heal Shame** for more tools for transforming guilt.

Communicate Your Needs

A baby is born with a need to be loved – and never outgrows it.

~ *Frank A. Clark*

Most people have a difficult time expressing their needs effectively and often revert to manipulation or reaction when attempting to have their needs met. Often an inability to effectively express one's needs is a result of learning ineffective communication strategies from our parents throughout our childhood and adolescence. As well, we may have learned to not express our needs for fear of looking too demanding or even for fear of being rejected.

When our needs are not met, because of failure to express them effectively, we can often go into various reactions: accumulating frustration and stress, depression, creating false ideas about not being loved or exploding with anger. Many of these reactions create strain on the relationship and can have partners feeling uncomfortable with these emotional states and can contribute to emotional withdrawal, fear and confusion. Unfortunately, when we hold back expression of our needs, we often create the very situation we try to avoid.

The benefit to learning to express your needs is that you and your partner may actually get your needs met. Relationships are richer and more peaceful when everyone feels supported to safely and honestly express their needs. When there is peace, your relationship flourishes. You both have the right to express your needs; the key is to learn to do it in a loving and effective way.

Finding a way to communicate your needs is very important when you are pregnant. Not only will it help your partner and/or support team meet your needs, but it will also give you the opportunity to relinquish control and let yourself be assisted. This will enable you to set aside some of your worries and focus more on your well being.

The basics of shifting to a relationship where your needs and the other person's needs are met entails:

Responsibility - If you are not getting your needs met, it is a starting point to realize that you may not have learned how to effectively and non-violently express your needs. You are the only one who can make this shift for yourself. Once you learn how to express your needs, you can invite your partner to learn, if they are willing.

Learning - Effective communication skills are learned skills, just like one learns to drive a car or bake a cake. There are certain steps that are required to ensure effective communication:

- **Understand family patterns and conditioning.** How did your parents and your partner's parents influence the ways you communicate?
- **Allow for a cooling off period.** A better time to resolve issues and effectively communicate is often when you are calm. When anger is present it can sabotage the process. If possible take the time to calm down and reflect on what you need.
- **Avoid speaking what you don't want.** Many people operate in

reaction mode and express what they don't want, rather than what their needs are. For example, instead of saying, "I don't like when you don't call me when you are working late." Trying saying: *When you work late and don't give me notice, dinner gets cold. I prefer that you call me when you know you are going to be working late. Would you be willing to call me earlier in the day?*

- **Avoid speaking in code.** Sometimes people speak in code to each other and expect the other person to telepathically know what they are talking about or even worse to magically know ahead of time what to do to meet their needs. For example, instead of saying, "Why can't you just love me?" Try saying: *I have a need to cuddle in the mornings and go for romantic walks in the evenings. I feel closer to you when we connect. Would you be willing to share those activities with me?* Often emotional reactions occur because we know we have a need that is not being met. However, we are not fully conscious of what that need is, but we expect the other person to know it and meet it for us.

- **Let go of manipulation.** Some people have learned violent ways to communicate by making ultimatums or using guilt or shame to change their partner's behavior. If you find yourself saying, "If you don't do ____, I am going to do ____", you are manipulating another. Change your behavior if you hear yourself reacting to a situation with statements like, "You make me sad" or "I hate myself because you do ____" or "If only you were a better person."

- **Refrain from attacks.** Ensure you are communicating fairly by not bringing in old arguments, swearing, name-calling and blaming. If you find yourself attacking another (or yourself) take responsibility and apologize as soon as possible. Attacks are like daggers into the heart of another. Unfortunately it destroys relationships. If you use this as a strategy, reflect on why you believe that you need to bully or cause harm to another. Is there a need that you want to express?

- **Distinguish between your wants versus your needs.** You may have a need to be acknowledged by your partner. However, having to do everything together in your free time may only be a want. Or in practical terms, you may have a need to get to the airport. But you want your partner to drive you there. Someone else may be able to drive you or you can take a taxi or public transportation.

- **Realize that your partner may not be able to meet all of your needs.** People often think that their partner has to meet all their emotional needs. In reality, we are all doing the best we can. It may be more effective to include others in your life to assist you to have your needs met. For example, a sibling, friend or parent may be available in ways your partner is not. Also, be open to friends and family being there to meet some of your partner's needs. It is healthy for couples to have outside friendships and activities that meet their overall needs.

- **Listen.** Effective and respectful listening requires you to refrain from interrupting. Focus your attention on what the other person is saying rather than thinking about what your next response will be. Once you've listened, mirror back what your partner has expressed to see if you understood them completely. If your partner says, "Stop interrupting me." Instead of reacting with defensiveness, you can say, "I hear you have a need for me to listen to you." When your partner feels heard, they feel safe to be more available to you.

- **Brainstorm your needs.** Take the time to reflect on what your needs actually are. Write them down and brainstorm to see what you learn about yourself.

Patience - Resolve to do what it takes to learn how to express your needs and to implement the necessary changes, even if it means you are a novice for a few months. Practice, practice, practice!

Reciprocity - Learning to communicate your needs is also about becoming aware that others may not have the skills to communicate their needs to you. This awareness is a key to being present for people and establishing a dialogue to assess the needs of others and guide them into non-violent communication of their needs. Establish a 'win-win' model of communication. What is your goal for your relationship? How can you also learn listen to and meet the needs of your partner without discarding or ignoring your needs?

Establishing a communication protocol - Establish an effective system of communicating with values of respect and love. Use a talking stick to learn to have one speaker at a time. I recommend that you keep the following suggestions in mind:

1. *Examine your thoughts.* Before you even start to communicate your needs, ensure that you search your mind and heart to be clear on what you need. Also think about your objective. Is there anything that you are trying to accomplish when you are communicating your needs? If so, what is it and how important is it?

2. *Be direct and honest.* Although others may be more than happy to help you, they can become frustrated if you choose to use indirect language and are not 100% honest. Make sure that you clearly tell people what you need without being cryptic, wishy-washy, manipulative or vague. Saying you will go to a dinner party when what you really want is to sleep will only create issues later that night. Make sure that you are clear about what you need in order to avoid

any misunderstandings.

3. *Ask in a positive manner.* Avoid demanding others meet your needs. Always ask in a positive manner. Use phrases such as, "I would appreciate it if you could…" or "Would you be willing to…" or "I have a need for…"

4. *Be grateful.* Finally, express gratitude and celebrate successful communication. Be sure that the people who are helping you are aware of how much you appreciate them. A simple thank you or even a thank you card will let them know just how much their thoughtfulness meant to you.

Communicating your needs can be a positive experience. If you find that people respond to you with irritation, frustration or anger, they may be a mirror for how ineffective your communication is with them. Review the section called "Use Non-Violent Communication" for more information on communicating compassionately.

Develop a Support Team of Friends & Family

Friends can help each other. A true friend is someone who lets you have total freedom to be yourself - and especially to feel. Or, not feel. Whatever you happen to be feeling at the moment is fine with them. That's what real love amounts to - letting a person be what he really is.

~Jim Morrison

Having a supportive team of friends and family in place is a blessing to your prenatal experience, as it provides an essential sense of community for you, your partner and your baby. Expecting   parents need to know that they have

70

people they can rely on for prenatal support during the birth of their baby and when they become new parents.

A baby is a blessing to all of existence. It is even said that all of nature rejoices in the birth of a baby. When you are expecting, you offer family and friends the opportunity to support you physically and emotionally in addition to sharing the adventure and joy. Support can also come in the form of having someone to discuss ideas with, drive you to an appointment, go to a prenatal yoga class with, share your concerns, enjoy a good laugh or go for daily walks.

When it comes to your birthing experience you may decide to have a few or many friends and family to support you during your experience or you may decide to just have your partner present. Whatever you decide, make sure you communicate your needs and plans ahead of time so everyone knows what to expect. You can also choose one person to communicate your needs to others who may be in attendance.

Remember, although most friends and family are excited to be of assistance during a pregnancy or birthing experience, some may not be available or suitable to support you in the way you most need. Look for the following qualities before you ask for help:

1. *They want to help*. In theory, most people would like to help especially if they are asked. However, when challenges arise some may either complain or will disappear when you need the help. Choose people you intuitively feel will have the commitment to follow through.

2. *They have the time and ability to help*. Even with the best intentions, some people just don't have the time, ability or

competence to help you.

3. *You can be at ease with them.* Ensure your support team is filled with people you can be yourself with, even when you are emotional or overcome with stress. For example, an expecting woman may have a mother-in-law who wants to be a support person. However, if their relationship is not close, any discomfort between them can create tension and unnecessary stress. A simple solution to honor the generosity of a mother-in-law that you are not close with is to ask her to help you by helping and supporting your partner.

4. *They get along with others.* When you choose your support team, make sure that everyone has a mutual rapport with each other. Taking on the role of a referee between supports will leave you feeling exhausted, overwhelmed and unsupported.

Make Social Connections With Other Moms to Be

We're connected, as women. It's like a spider web. If one part of that web vibrates,
if there's trouble, we all know it, but most of the time we're just too scared,
or selfish, or insecure to help. But if we don't help each other, who will?

~ Sarah Addison Allen, The Peach Keeper

Developing a social connection with other expecting women is a key element in maternal health. Studies have found that women who experience high levels of community were healthier than those without social connections.[20] A lack of connection can leave women feeling unsupported and disconnected. Creating a support network with other expecting women is important for:

- Emotional support
- Education
- Meeting new friends
- Creating a support network
- Learning about events
- Sharing experiences
- Sharing referrals
- Helping others

Most cities and towns offer opportunities and events for expecting women to connect. If your neighborhood is lacking a meet up for expecting moms, then consider starting one in your area. Some great places to meet other expecting moms include:

- Meetup.com - just search for "moms to be" or "first-time pregnant moms"
- Online forums and support groups
- Prenatal yoga and fitness classes
- Prenatal courses

Find Professional Prenatal Support

A mother does not become pregnant in order to provide employment to medical people.
Giving birth is an ecstatic jubilant adventure not available to males.
It is a woman's crowning creative experience of a lifetime.

~ John Stevenson

A great way for you to feel relaxed and confident about your pregnancy is to find professional prenatal health practitioners who are knowledgeable about pregnancy health, fetal development and birthing. Health practitioners with prenatal expertise can assist you to enjoy your pregnancy and have a safe and more peaceful birthing experience.

Prenatal practitioners could include prenatal coaches, Hypnobirthing coaches, Hypnobabies instructors, herbalists, acupuncturists, nutritionists, nurses, doctors, midwives or doulas. Look for professionals who are compassionate, experienced with great references and who respect and support your needs.

If you find that your visits with your prenatal practitioner are stressful and uncomfortable, feel free to find someone new. Find one who will support your prenatal care and shares your views on childbirth. Just like in any situation, not everyone is a perfect match.

Start by asking other expecting moms or new moms for recommendations. Always ensure that the person you choose is someone that you are comfortable with, fits your budget, has the time to listen to your concerns and is understanding of your fears and beliefs.

Visit a Therapist or Counselor

I love therapy! There's nothing like talking to someone
who has no emotional tie to your life.

~*Eva Mendes*

Finding a professional to assist you to understand your issues and concerns can be a beneficial way to enhance self-growth, heal interpersonal relationships, get a clearer perspective on life, prevent or eliminate behaviors or psychological symptoms like anxiety or depression, heal emotional conflicts, strengthen spiritual growth, learn helpful strategies or improve mental health.

Along the spectrum of counseling, there are many options including counselors, clinical counselors, family therapists, pastors, priests, spiritual teachers, traditional psychologists, psychiatrists, energy psychologists, EFT practitioners, nutritionists and emotional coaches.

A major difference between a psychiatrist and all other counseling practitioners is that psychiatrists are medical doctors who are authorized to prescribe drugs and order brain-imaging studies. Typically they are trained in assessing, diagnosing, treating and preventing mental illness.

Some counselors handle any area of concern, but many tend to specialize in a specific counseling niche such as marriage, anxiety, addictions, phobias, postpartum, family, anger management, etc.

Group counseling is also a great way to overcome stress. They are less formal than other types of therapy and they allow you to participate at your own level of comfort. If you are not confident with sharing, then you can sit back and learn from others' sharing.

If clinical forms of therapy are not for you, there are effective non-clinical counselors and health practitioners that may be able to assist you to clear emotional conflicts and relieve stress and anxiety. Some of the many options include:

- Neuro-Linguistic Programming (NLP)
- Emotional Freedom Technique (EFT)
- Emotions Coaching
- Art Therapy
- Intuitive Healing
- Thought Field Therapy (TFT)

- Spiritual Counseling
- Pre & Perinatal Somatic Therapy

If you need assistance, seek help early in your pregnancy to ensure any emotional conflicts, anxieties or issues are resolved so you can enjoy a peaceful pregnancy.

Find a Helpful Support Group

Individually, we are one drop. Together, we are an ocean.

~ *Ryunosuke Satoro*

Having a healthy support system is important for preventing, managing and overcoming stress before, during and after your pregnancy. Whether or not you have friends and family to support you, you can find additional support through the use of support groups. A support group is simply a group of people who meet to share thoughts, experiences and information. Everyone in the group is there for each other to provide a safe place to share issues or to learn from experiences.

At one time, support groups were limited to meeting halls or places where people could connect in person. Over the years, it has grown to meet the needs of a variety of situations and many support groups can now be found on the Internet. The available spectrum of support groups include:

- *Traditional Support Groups* - These are groups where you meet people who have the same interests or concerns as you. It is usually done on a regular basis and has a support leader who facilitates the meetings each week.

- *Networks* - These are groups that bring people together so they can help each other overcome a specific problem. They usually have one focus.

- *Online Communities* - A great way to experience support is to join an online prenatal community. Typically these groups offer webinars and teleseminars, forums, discussion groups or news groups. Yahoo, Google and Facebook have a range of prenatal communities with valuable information and inspiration.

As you can see, there are many different places for you to find a support group but it is important to look for a few key factors in your support group. Healthy support groups:

- *Have organization.* Although support groups can be informal, it is better to find a support group that offers both an organized framework and regular meetings. They should be organized and group members should know what is expected at a meeting.

- *Are encouraging to all members.* Along with organization, make sure that your support group is fair and inclusive.

- *Have similar interests or fill a specific need.* Make sure any support group you join is geared towards your needs so you can find the emotional support you are looking for.

Hire a Doula

Asking your husband to be your sole guide through labor is like asking him to lead the way on a climb of Mt Everest. He may be smart and trustworthy, you may love him, but in the Himalayas you'd both be a lot better off with a Sherpa!

~ Pam England

Historically, continuous support during birthing has been provided throughout time by other women. It has only been within the last 100 years that continuous support has been overlooked. Today there is a resurgence of women asking other women, such as friends, family or a doula, to be there to support them and their partner throughout their birthing.

A doula is a birthing partner who provides non-medical, continuous support for the mother and her family during the various stages of birthing and delivery. The word 'doula' is an ancient Greek word meaning "a woman who serves." She is a valuable resource who can help relieve stress before, during and after delivery.

Research studies have found that doula care during birth is associated with a reduction of the duration of the birthing process, the use of pain medication, childbirth interventions and cesarean deliveries.[21] In addition, research shows that doula support improves childbirth outcomes for the mom and baby, increases timely initiation of breastfeeding,[22] increases positive maternal feelings about the childbirth experience, reduces postpartum depression[23] and assists parents to feel more confident, secure and cared for during and after their birthing experience.

According to DONA, a doula's key roles[24] are to:

- Recognize birth as a key life experience that the mother will remember all her life.
- Understand the physiology of birth and the emotional needs of a woman in labor.
- Assist the woman and her partner in preparing for and carrying out their plans for the birth.
- Stay by the side of the laboring woman throughout the entire labor.
- Provide emotional support, physical comfort measures, an objective viewpoint and assistance to the woman in getting the information she needs to make good decisions.
- Facilitate communication between the laboring woman, her partner and clinical care providers.
- Perceive her role as one who nurtures and protects the woman's memory of her birth experience.
- Allow the woman's partner to participate at his/her comfort level

If you have not considered it yet, I recommend that you hire a doula to help you during the birth of your baby. Doulas offer many prenatal services as well: offering suggestions on caring for yourself and your growing baby, listening to prenatal concerns, helping you make your birth plan and educating you on birthing so you know what to expect.

During the birthing phase, professional doulas use techniques such as patterned breathing, massage, acupressure and imagery to reduce a woman's pain. They know helpful position changes to accelerate the birthing process or aid in fetal positioning. Doulas offer guidance and encouragement to minimize fear and anxiety and encourage communication and loving touch between the birthing woman and her partner.

After delivery, you can hire a postpartum doula to come for a few visits to ensure your postpartum needs are met and your transition into parenthood is smoother. Postpartum doulas assist with support, some newborn care, meal preparation and light household cleaning. They also offer education on coping skills for new parents, breastfeeding and physical recovery from birth. When necessary doulas will suggest referrals for further postpartum support.

When you look for a doula, consider the following to make the best choice for you and your family:

1. **Set up an interview with a number of doulas.** Remember that you and your partner need to feel comfortable with the doula prior to the birthing to avoid feeling uncomfortable during the birthing process. Interview several doulas to find the one you feel most connected with.

2. **Ensure that the doula has the education and credentials that you are comfortable with.** Doulas who are certified with a national doula organization are available. However, there are experienced doulas that have chosen to not certify and are just as qualified. If certification is important to you, ask to see their credentials or references. Sometimes the best qualifications are revealed in the experience and client references that a doula has from previous births.

3. **Check their availability.** Make sure that you hire a doula who can offer continuous support throughout your pregnancy, during the birth and into postpartum. Ask if they have a backup doula to fill in for them if they happen to be unavailable to attend your birth.

Schedule an appointment with the backup doula so you are sure you feel comfortable with her as well.

4. **Inquire about the fees.** Make sure that you ask about the fees, payment schedule and ask what the refund policy is if the doula is not able to attend your birth.

5. **Listen to your intuition when choosing a doula.** The most important element is that you feel comfortable with your doula.

After you choose a doula, ask plenty of questions, express your needs, voice your fears about delivery and also go over any concerns that you may have with having a doula attend the birth. By being open, you will find that the doula can address your needs and alleviate the fears and stress you are feeling regarding the upcoming delivery.

In addition to professional doulas, caring female relatives or friends with some training as a doula or those who have had their own positive experience birthing can also enhance the birth and postpartum experience.

Join a Prenatal Class

When you know better you do better.

~ Maya Angelou

Prenatal classes offer empowering opportunities for expecting parents to learn about fetal development, birthing options, the birthing process, pain management during childbirth and also infant care. There are a variety of prenatal classes including Hypnobabies, Hypnobirthing, Lamaze, the Bradley

Method, Pre and Perinatal Somatic Therapy and Dancing for Birth.

Research studies have reported that prenatal education courses assist expecting moms to alleviate anxiety, put their concerns at ease and contribute to the bonding they have with their baby.[25] Prenatal classes are designed to prepare new parents for the road ahead. Whether it is your first pregnancy or you're an experienced mom, the classes are a wonderful way to unwind, bond with your partner, connect with other expecting parents and learn emerging information on birthing.

Avoid Micromanaging Your Pregnancy

Change your focus, and you change your level of happiness.

~Anthony Robbins

While mindfulness is a healthy practice, micromanaging is exhausting and stressful, especially during a pregnancy. Learn to do the best you can and let go of the need to have a 'perfect' pregnancy. Instead focus on having a peaceful and balanced pregnancy. Ask yourself, "What can I do today or in this moment to take care of my needs and the needs of my baby?"

Micromanaging can be a symptom of an emotional issue, such as fear of the unknown. You have a choice of whether to feed fear or cultivate peace. Let go of the idea that everything needs to be controlled. If you are susceptible to obsessing about your pregnancy and are stuck in a stressful situation, there are some tools and activities that can assist you to change the thought patterns in your brain.

Shift your focus by orienting yourself to activities that cultivate joy and relaxation, wellness, aliveness and peace of mind. Journaling, taking time to catch up on your reading, learning to cook healthy meals, walking or swimming can help take your attention from micromanaging your pregnancy. Asking for help and letting others assist with household tasks, work or planning your birth is another way to let go of control over your pregnancy.

✓ Learn Emotional Freedom Technique (review the section called "Use Emotional Freedom Technique") to release trapped emotions and obsessive behavioral patterns. Tap with a phrase like: "Even though I feel compelled to micromanage my pregnancy, I fully and completely love and accept myself" or "Even though I feel afraid of the unknown, I fully and completely love and accept myself."

If your obsessions or stress are unmanageable seek out professional help from prenatal and/or mental health practitioners as early as possible in your pregnancy.

Resolve Conflicts With Friends or Family

Families are like fudge - mostly sweet with a few nuts.

~Author Unknown

Going into your pregnancy, it is important to assess your relationships and resolve outstanding conflicts to release unnecessary stress that may affect you and your baby. Many families have some kind of issue or emotional strain between two or more family members. If the conflict is resolvable, there are a few tips that you should remember:

• *Take responsibility.* It takes courage to take the first step in peaceful resolution. Identify your role in the conflict or how you contributed to the situation by becoming aware of your perceptions and reactions. By doing this, you give yourself the power to find a solution.

- *Invite resolution.* Reach out to the other person and invite them to participate in the resolution of the conflict.

- *Stay calm.* Always approach the conflict in a calm manner. If you are unable to be calm, find a way to get your points across without being combative. This could be waiting until you have calmed down enough, asking someone to work as a mediator or writing down your points before you approach conflict resolution.

- *Be aware of your feelings.* Before you go into conflict resolution, be aware of how you feel and find ways to ground your emotions. If you find that you are overwhelmed by emotions when you go to resolve the problem, have someone there to support you. If you feel like crying let the tears flow.

- *Listen to the other person.* Although you may have a number of things you want to say, it is important to let the other person have an opportunity to share their side. When they speak, listen rather than thinking about what your response is going to be to ensure you really hear what they are sharing and so they feel fully heard.

- *Use 'I' statements.* Once it is your turn to talk, use 'I' statements. Phrases such as, "I feel," or "I thought." This makes it less combative and will open up the other person to hearing what you are saying. Communicate your needs and feelings in an honest, non-violent way.

- *Find a win-win resolution.* Once you have talked through how both of you are feeling, work with the other person to come up with a resolution. Identify specific solutions to meet each other's needs or preferences.

- *Own up to your mistakes.* Whenever you have been in the wrong, make sure you own up to your mistakes. Apologize for your mistakes and be heartfelt about it.

- *Choose to forgive.* Holding on to past grievances creates stress within you. Allow yourself the gift of forgiving others and yourself.

- *Know when to cut your losses.* Although we all want to believe that every conflict can be resolved, there are some that just can't or some that take more than one effort to resolve. If the confrontation becomes mean spirited or abusive or if you find that you have reached an impasse, calmly state that it can't be solved at this time and disengage. It is better to leave before it becomes even more difficult to correct.

- *Do something fun with the person you've been at odds with.* Sometimes healing happens when you can just allow yourself to enjoy the other person's company.

Avoid Negative People

You are worthy of happiness, health, success and love. You deserve to have good friends, fulfilling personal relationships, and strong family bonds.

~*Jane Powell*

In addition to building a support team with your family and friends and eliminating sources of stress, it is also important to stop spending time with negative and angry people. I know a few people who love to complain and gossip, and no matter how much I try to steer them toward positive conversations, they always bring the conversation back to negative talk. If I spend time with them, I notice my mood and thoughts become affected, and I can even slip into negative talk if I am not mindful.

Stress from negative interactions with others can have an affect on your mental and physical health leaving you feeling stressed, anxious, fearful, angry, annoyed or frustrated. Experiencing these stressful states can have negative consequences on the health of both you and your baby.

There are some well-meaning people who may even want to help you by sharing their negative points of view and experiences about pregnancy and birthing. Discern which information and suggestions are helpful without taking things personally. You can also be clear with others that you are only interested in hearing constructive talk regarding pregnancy and childbirth.

Some effective strategies include:
- Reflect on how you contribute to negative interactions and figure out what you can do to change your behavior.

- Be clear with your self about what is acceptable and unacceptable behavior. We teach others how to treat us. Be clear and honest about what kinds of conversations you are open to participating in.
- Decrease the amount of time you spend with negative people.
- When necessary, phase negative people out of your life.
- Learn how to communicate non-violently.
- Stop taking things personally. People who attack others do so because there are emotional conflicts within them. Understanding their behavior with compassion allows you to see that it isn't about you.
- Let people be. If someone is negative, let them be negative. You don't have to change them. That is their business. Take responsibility for your state of mind, thoughts, emotions and actions.
- Establish new positive relationships.
- Nourish healthy relationships with positive people.

Let Go of Taking Things Personally

Whatever happens around you, don't take it personally...
Nothing other people do is because of you. It is because of themselves.

~ Miguel Ruiz, The Four Agreements

Do you ever find yourself taking things personally? Do you feel hurt or offended by the actions or remarks of others? A great deal of stress and frustration could be eliminated just from the act of learning how to not take things personally. Unfortunately for many people who take things personally, it is a learned behavior of agreeing with another's point of view or projecting their own belief about themselves on another. Either way, people who take things personally have a low sense of themselves.

If someone says to you, "What a b#@$%" and you take it personally, you have bought into their belief of who you are. Instead, free yourself from the influence of the other, by first identifying who you truly are and second by seeing that others have their own lack of self-esteem regardless of how aggressive they seem.

Others

How others behave has little to do with you. Everyone experiences life differently and expresses themselves from the way they perceive and respond to their environment based on the lessons they learned about themselves and others from our caregivers and early life experiences. These lessons and experiences become the template by which people measure their self-worth and capacity to be empathic, caring and genuine.

I know some people who enjoy putting others down or complaining about everything. At the root of their complaining is deep suffering caused by unresolved emotional conflicts that have been present their entire lifetime, often since childhood.

In response to the initial emotional conflicts they experienced, one of their strategies may be to use negativity as a lens to view the world in a way to 'safely' anticipate disappointment. They may also use the strategy of being strongly attached to ideas of how things should or shouldn't be. For the most part, no matter what their experience, until they heal the conflict at the root of their suffering, they will always see things from a negative slant. These types of people may have experienced tremendous disappointment and may have been disciplined strongly as children. Most of the time, people who are negative are not conscious that they are negative.

Overly Sensitive People

People who tend to take things personally also have a strategy to see the world from their point of view. If you have this tendency, you may hear your self saying, "Why does this always happen to me?" Or "How come my brother always attacks me?" The person you are reacting to may not even be behaving in a negative way. If you have a pattern of taking things personally, you could be seeing others actions tainted through a lens of negativity.

I am very close with a person who tends to think that everyone is putting her down by their every word and action. She even thinks when people share their successes it is an attempt to put her down. Although this is an extreme version of a highly reactive and blaming person on the surface, it gives us a clear example of how the milder reactivity can taint our beliefs. At the root of this woman's suffering is that she values herself as less than everyone else. However, self-devaluation is not always an easy thing for the conscious mind to take, so it projects the role onto another person. Although the other person may not be attacking, the ego will filter every word and action through a self-devaluating lens, making it appear as though "others believe they are better than me."

Taking things personally can also sabotage your relationship with your partner or spouse. For example, when your partner doesn't do something you want them to do, the self-sabotaging ego then labels the action or inaction as a sign that, "He doesn't love me." At the root of the situation is a belief that "I am not loveable." Essentially, what another person does or doesn't do for us is never a sign of whether they love us or not. Nor is it a healthy way to measure self worth.

Strategies

Whether you are being negative or they are being negative, or you're both being negative, here are some strategies for resolving your situation:

- ✓ Let go of your expectations and judgments of others.

- ✓ Feel compassion for negative people. Try to understand the suffering they may be experiencing.

- ✓ Feel compassion for yourself.

- ✓ Allow yourself to be free of the influence of others. Just say, "I choose to be free from what that person says or does."

- ✓ Find ways to be free of your own thoughts around what others might be thinking or why they might be behaving. You could say, "I choose to be free from what I think this person might be saying."

- ✓ Break the habit of the negative mind by finding a positive way to respond. For example, if you've been triggered, be truly grateful and use the situation as an opportunity to address what needs to be healed within you.

- ✓ Ask yourself, "How can this issue get any better than this?"

- ✓ Clarify what you have heard from another by mirroring what they've said and by asking them if you've heard them correctly.

- ✓ Express how you feel to the other person using non-violent communication. For example, "When you say _____, I feel sad and angry. Would you be willing to refrain from saying _____?"

You cannot control what others do, however you can reflect on and change how you respond to situations.

Cultivate a Flexible Mind

The green reed which bends in the wind is stronger
than the mighty oak which breaks in a storm.

~ Confucius

Do you have a habit of using words like "always" or "never"? Do you hear yourself saying, "You never listen to me" or "My mother never loved me"? Do you notice yourself thinking that things have to be a certain way?

Whether you have a tendency to be inflexible all the time or once in a while, rigid thinking is limited thinking and can create situations of stress within our own mind when relating to others and when faced with challenges.

Rigid thinking has its roots in early childhood experiences of real or perceived unmet needs, lack of safety and/or abandonment. When faced with these traumas, emotional survival strategies and defense mechanisms develop. One of these strategies is rigid thinking, as it develops out of the need for a safe place by creating unbending, already-formulated beliefs and pre-accepted opinions.

The Benefits of a Flexible Mind

There are many emotional and behavioral benefits to cultivating an agile and flexible mind. Some of the best advantages of a flexible mind are:

- ✓ Creative thinking

- ✓ Access to more information and potential solutions

- ✓ Inclusive thinking

- ✓ Healthier relationships

- ✓ A sense of freedom and peace

- ✓ Adaptability

- ✓ Effective problem solving

- ✓ Less stress

- ✓ Knowing when to be rigid and when to be flexible

Strategies

When others suggest you are inflexible or you observe yourself thinking or saying statements that are rigid and unbending, reflect on what is at the root of your inflexibility.

- Are there any emotional, physical or psychological needs not being met?
- Are there fears at the root of your inflexibility?
- Can you identify, express and release your emotions around your thinking?
- Are you willing to see things differently? Are you willing to choose new experiences that are different from how you normally interact with the world?

While some people have learned very early how to be flexible and seem to be naturally more laid back, flexibility can also be intentionally developed. Here are some strategies and ways to develop flexible thinking:

- ✓ Use Emotional Freedom Technique to clear rigid beliefs that are tied in with perceptions, experiences, fears and past traumas. (See the section called "Use Emotional Freedom Technique.")

- ✓ If you normally demand something be done in a particular way invite the other person to do it their way.

- ✓ Change your regular routine. Take a new route to work. Pick up a book from a genre you normally wouldn't read.

- ✓ Try something new. Try a different flavor of ice cream or introduce a new healthy food into your diet. Take up a new hobby.

- ✓ Change your environment. Go somewhere you've never been. Eat your lunch somewhere new. Visit an area of town you've never been.

- ✓ Observe how others respond to situations. Who seems to be more relaxed and more peaceful? Learn from them.

- ✓ Refrain from using words like "always" and "never" when describing how others behave.

- ✓ Learn healthy communication skills (review the section called "Use Non-Violent Communication").

Negative Thinking vs. Positive Thinking

The state of your life is nothing more than a reflection of your state of mind.

~ Dr. Wayne W. Dyer

Do you see the glass as half full or half empty? Do you experience negative or peaceful internal dialogues? If you have ever experienced negative thinking and emotional states, you know how challenging it can be to shift out of those experiences. If a person does not actively seek to transform negativity, it can sabotage a person's whole life contributing to difficulties in relationships, self esteem, physical and mental health, work and the direction of their life path.

Negativity is damaging, corrupting and causes stress. It contributes to insomnia and depression, destroys relationships, affects self esteem, shortens your life, affects other people, creates a victim mentality, compounds challenging issues and programs your mind. Negativity can show up as feeling bad about yourself, your situation or the future. There are many manifestations of negativity in people that range from being a violent person to being a drama queen and even to being a victim.

Through my coaching practice I have worked with many people who used negativity to keep people from getting close to them. They feared rejection so deeply that they rejected the other person first, to prevent inevitable rejection in the end. It is a profound self-sabotage that begins early in life as a survival strategy. However, it no longer serves and must be changed if a meaningful and peaceful life is to be experienced.

What causes negativity?

- **Diet** – What you eat has a profound affect on your brain functioning and your emotional and mental health. Deficiencies of vitamin, minerals, essential fatty acids and proteins affect your state of mind. Key food items to include in your diet are dark leafy greens, quinoa, fresh fish, eggs, avocado, coconut oil, vegetables, fruits, nuts and seeds. For example, when I don't eat enough greens I experience frustration and agitation in my brain. Junk foods can also change your mood, resulting in agitation and negativity.

- **Foods Additives** – MSG, aspartame, glutamate, stabilizers, preservatives and chemicals in processed foods can also contribute to negative mental states by changing hormones and damaging nerve cells. I once had a terrible chemical reaction to theatre popcorn. Until my body processed the chemicals, my symptoms included agitation, confusion and obsessive-compulsive behavior. After doing some research I found out that the flavor enhancing chemicals they add to the popcorn damages nerve cells and disrupts hormones.

- **Dehydration** – Even when mildly dehydrated, cellular stress contributes to degraded mood, headaches, lower concentration and difficulty completing tasks.

- **The Environment** – Environmental exposures to mold, pesticides, heavy metals and other chemicals can disrupt our hormones and neurotransmitters. Also, what you read, watch and hear affects your mood.

- **Limiting Beliefs** – If you have a negative attitude it may be because you have false beliefs about life in general or specific areas of it. To make a shift in mood, shift your beliefs and attitudes.

- **Infectious Organisms** – Certain viruses and bacteria can affect our hormones and can even impair or damage the brain.

- **Negative People** – Birds of a feather flock together! If you want to be more positive, spend time with those who are positive.

- **Hormones** – Hormonal fluctuations and deficiencies or excess levels of certain hormones can affect mood.

- **Feeling Powerless** – Feeling like you have no control over your destiny can be crippling. Take responsibility for your life and design it to nourish you, even if it means taking one small step each day.

- **Unmet Needs** – The stress of your needs not being met contributes to negativity. The key to having your needs met is to understand what they are and to communicate them effectively.

As damaging as negativity is, it can be transformed and healing of the body and mind are possible. The benefits of thinking positively are abundant including an improved mood, more energy, healthier body and brain, experiencing joy and peace, healthier relationships and opening to love and gratitude. Positive thinking programs the mind to see opportunities, to be aware of the larger picture and to attract positive experiences.

How to Change a Negative Mindset

✓ *Focus on what you want.* I recommend that you take some time to reflect on what you would like to create in every area of your life. If you aren't sure, brainstorm the possibilities. Having a personal vision inspires the mind with a positive focus.

✓ *Connect with your emotions.* If you are feeling stressed, angry, annoyed, anxious or depressed, ask your self, "Why?" What is at the root of these emotional states?

✓ *Acknowledge your negative thoughts.* As negative thoughts arise, observe them and let them go. You may even want to say "all clear" each time a negative thought pops up and then move on.

✓ *Separate the negative from the positive.* Identify the negative thoughts that are linked to negative emotions such as jealousy, worry or disappointment. Once you know which thoughts are negative, you can begin to deal with them.

✓ *Replace negative thoughts for positive.* The brain is elastic and malleable to change. Begin training your brain to see the positive. It may be that you have to ask your self, "What are the positives of this situation?" If you are worried about the health of your baby, think about the miraculous growth of your baby or take the time to smile from your heart to your baby. By committing your attention to see the positive in everything, you are telling your brain to look for it. If you do this for a minimum of 45 days, you will notice how quickly your mindset changes.

✓ *Develop an attitude of gratitude.* Be grateful for what you have in your life. Spend 30 seconds or more each morning and night expressing five things for which you are grateful. Every time you eat a meal, say thank you to nature. Every time you see a person smile, say thank you inside. Say thank you to every cell in your body for doing a great job.

✓ *Be kind to your self and others.* Let go of past mistakes and learn from your mistakes. Have a loving attitude toward all people, especially you.

✓ *Stop trying to predict the future.* Let go of trying to figure out what is going to happen or investing in future possibilities. When you focus on potential negative outcomes, you can very easily attract them. If you have fears, acknowledge them without dwelling on them. If you are going to fantasize about the future, why not visualize positive outcomes instead.

- **Avoid blaming and complaining.** If you find yourself blaming someone else or complaining about something else, drop and give me ten push-ups! ☺ Just joking. Instead find ten things or people to compliment or say something positive about.

- **Avoid using negative generalizations.** Words such as "always," "never," "every time," "everyone" and "no one" only limit your thinking and pigeon hole other people. Be aware of how positive or negative your language is throughout the day.

- **Be open to new possibilities.** Many people walk around with preconceived ideas about how things are or how they should be. Expecting moms do this with their pregnancies, births and their preconceived ideas of motherhood. Look at your prenatal journey as an adventure filled with interesting experiences and positive possibilities you now get to experience.

Avoid Crowded Places

Honk if you hate noise pollution.

~ From a bumper sticker, author unknown

Between the noise, pressure and energetic bustle of crowded places, city life has been found to affect the brain in adverse ways. Residents of densely populated urban areas have higher rates of mental illness, anxiety, and urban stress than those of country dwellers due to increased incidences of being on guard, social activity and hyperactivity of the brain.[26]

Some people thrive among large groups of people, while many people feel drained by them. Crowds can affect our mood and behavior and can magnify the way we feel and react. Unless you are one of those people who feed off of other people's energy, I suggest avoiding crowded places, such as concerts, Saturday afternoon at the grocery store or driving home during rush hour.

Learn About the Benefits of Natural Birthing

Keeping active during labour and adopting natural, upright or crouching birth positions is the safest, most enjoyable, most economical and sensible way for the majority of women to give birth.

~ Janet Balaskas

Birthing customs and rituals vary around the world and over time. Throughout recorded history, and most likely since women began giving birth, the common birthing position has been some form of upright position. The mid-seventeenth century ushered in the practice of having women lie down on their backs, as it was easier for the medical staff to use forceps. Even today with modern research, the knowledge of human physiology, experience and insights into gravity, it is a wonder that anyone would suggest that reclining on your back is a more effect way to give birth.

Yet western culture, throughout the last few centuries, has been following the ritual of placing birthing women into lying positions. Luckily for birthing women today, more and more health care practitioners are catching up with modern science to realize the benefits of natural birth and the use of sitting and squatting positions rather than the reclining position.

Lying Down Vs. Upright Positions

Research studies suggest that lying down to give birth slows down the birthing process and is more dangerous than an upright position.[27] [28] Researchers have found that the use of an upright position during the second stage of labor has many benefits compared to a lying on your back. Here are some known benefits of squatting:

- ✓ Gravity helps reduce the duration of the birthing process[29]

- ✓ Opens the pelvis 30% more than lying down[30]

- ✓ Allows the body to be in a position to move and rock

- ✓ Can help relieve the pain of back labor

- ✓ Decreases the need for the use of forceps[31]

- ✓ Helps shorten the pushing phase of birthing

✓ Decreases episiotomy rates[32]

✓ Reduced reporting of severe pain

✓ Fewer abnormal fetal heart rate patterns[33]

Chemical Interventions

Chemical interventions like epidurals can leave you emotional detached from your birthing experience. Some of the common side effects associated with epidurals are itching, slowed heart beat, shallow breathing, nausea, fever,[34] confusion and higher risk for instrumental vaginal delivery.[35] Since the drugs used in epidurals cross the placenta blood barrier the fetus also experiences a medicated state and the side effects of the drugs.

Epidurals can also contribute to fetal distress [36] by slowing down the second stage of birthing,[37] decelerating the fetal heart rate, [38] increasing antibiotic treatment for possible sepsis[39] and hindering the baby's ability to nurse[40] and bond with mom. Although studies suggest that epidural pharmaceuticals don't harm the baby very much, there is no research proving that anesthetic and narcotics don't harm the baby at all. There are no drugs that have proven to be safe for a baby in the womb.

High dose epidurals can also block the ability to feel if your bladder is full or to feel sensation in your legs, making it risky to even walk to the bathroom. This means a nurse will most likely insert a urinary catheter to drain urine. Having access to your legs during birth is essential to being able to walk around, squat and to transition into positions your body guides you into.

Due to the increased health risks of having an epidural, you'll also be hooked up to a fetal monitor and an IV. The IV is to give the medical team access to your veins in case your require emergency medications. It is also used to keep you hydrated since you will not be allowed to eat or drink after you have your epidural placed. Other potential risks associated with high dose epidurals include:

- Longer second stage labor and higher rates of episiotomy[41]
- Increased use of urinary catheters (which increases risk for urinary tract infections and need for antibiotics), IVs, monitoring devices and additional pharmacological intervention
- Non-existent, uneven or incomplete pain relief
- Unintentional dural puncture
- Post lumbar puncture headaches[42]
- An increased use of instruments and devices in vaginal delivery by as much as 20 times[43]
- Maternal hypotension and an increased risk of cesarean surgery by 2-3 times in first time mothers[44]
- Maternal inflammatory fever, which is associated with newborn blood infection, antibiotic treatment,[45] brain injury and learning deficits in later childhood[46]
- Increased intervention for fetal distress[47]
- Fetal bradycardia (an abnormally slow fetal heart rate)[48]
- Increased incidences of birth trauma for the newborn due to an increase in duration of labor and higher rates of instrument assisted deliveries and cesareans

The Risks Associated with Cesarean Surgeries

It is believed that cesarean births are on the rise due to the increased willingness of staff to follow a cesarean protocol,[49] scheduling convenience for the physician, professional fear of malpractice,[50] "designer births" or side effects of labor interventions. A number of short-term and long-term risks for the newborn that are associated with cesareans including persistent pulmonary hypertension,[51] altered postnatal responses and physiology (which may lead to disease later in life), impaired lung function, reduced body temperatures, altered metabolism, altered feeding, altered immune cell response and reduced blood pressure.

Children born by cesarean birth have a higher risk of being diagnosed with neurological issues, stress related problems, and immune related conditions such as asthma, chronic inflammation of the nose and sinuses, food allergy and type-I Diabetes.[52] Researchers have also found that elective cesarean surgeries had a 69% higher risk of neonatal mortality than planned vaginal deliveries.[53]

New research also suggests that a child's first exposure to bacteria occurs during the passage down the mother's vaginal canal. Children who are delivered by cesarean surgery miss this opportunity and have been found to lack beneficial bacteria called Bacteroides and Escherichia-Shigella compared to vaginally born infants.[54]

The recovery for a cesarean takes longer than a vaginal birth. The difficulties and risks for maternal health include pain, reduced mobility, abdominal wound problems and higher levels of uterine infection than women with assisted or spontaneous vagina birth.[55] In addition, uterine rupture risk increases with multiple cesarean surgeries.[56] For the health of you and your baby, whenever possible, reduce the risk of needing to have a cesarean birth by reducing stress during pregnancy, eating nutritious foods, utilizing the upright position during the birthing process, avoiding high dose epidurals and not opting for an elective cesarean surgery.

There are birthing situations that necessitate medical intervention. If you require a cesarean birth because of a high risk pregnancy or emergency situation, do what you can to ensure your needs and your baby's needs are taken care of with family support, continuous care with a doula and clear indication to medical staff of your wish to bond with your baby as soon as possible. After you have recovered from a cesarean, create opportunities to further bond with your baby. Have a heart-centered conversation with your newborn about what happened and how although you wished the birth went smoother, you are so happy that s/he is with you now.

Benefits of Natural Childbirth

Birthing naturally offers a woman the option of being fully present for her experience and her body. Many natural childbirth experts state that the sensations associated with contractions are natural and valuable in facilitating birth, as it guides women to find what positions or breathing feels best to alleviate pain. When a women's pain sensation is eliminated with medication, she is cut off from communication with her body. The birthing process may slow down and become less efficient.

In response to pain and stress, the body naturally produces pain-relieving hormones called endorphins. Unfortunately, when intense pain first surfaces, women often panic and become overcome with fear of additional pain, leading them to request narcotics or an epidural before the body has a chance to produce its own pain relief. If you have the ability to relax and surrender into the experience, these natural pain-relieving hormones will kick in.

There is growing evidence in research that strategies such as immersion in water, relaxation techniques, hypnotherapy, massage and acupuncture may relieve birthing pain and improve childbirth experience when compared with placebo or standard care. Relaxation and acupuncture are associated with fewer assisted vaginal births. Acupuncture is also associated with fewer caesarean surgeries.[57] Other birthing strategies that have been reported to contribute to increased relaxation and the reduction of pain and duration of birthing include yoga,[58] squatting, walking,[59] rocking, abdominal breathing, vocalizing, warm showers, acupressure, massage and reflexology.[60]

In vaginal births, researchers have discovered that babies delivered with the use of forceps or vacuum had higher levels of stress hormones,[61] higher rates of cephalohematomas, neonatal jaundice, scalp injuries and deaths.[62] Women are also at risk during instrumental deliveries for disease, perineal pain and lacerations, hematomas, blood loss, anemia and short and long-term urinary and fecal incontinence.[63]

Strategies for Natural Pain-Relief

Throughout your birthing experience, you can assist your body to produce endorphins and oxytocin with various strategies.

- ✓ Stay calm and relaxed.

- ✓ Be informed and learn relaxation techniques and natural pain management strategies by reading, watching videos or taking courses on natural childbirth methods such as Hypnobirthing, Hypnobabies, the Bradley Method or Lamaze.

- ✓ Stay upright and use gravity to assist you in birthing.

- ✓ Utilize massage or a warm bath for pain relief.

- ✓ Birth in a comfortable, private space free of disturbances and noise.

- ✓ Surround yourself with a supportive and positive birthing team who mindfully meets your needs.

- ✓ Avoid unnecessary procedures and epidural analgesia.

- ✓ Trust your body.

- ✓ Breathe.

It's About You & Your Baby

Regardless of the choices, strategies and environment you select for birthing, make them your own. Empower yourself to find comfort in the ways that work best for you. You have the opportunity to create a birthing experience to be the incredible transforming process it was meant to be.

Read books, watch videos and talk to a variety of women with varying experiences. Think about birthing not only from your perspective, but also from your baby's point of view. Reflect on what is best for your baby's experience of the event, as well as his or her future health and development. Envision your baby's first emergence, how would you like it to be?

Take a walk in your mind of all the current practices that tend to be used during birthing. What would each of them feel like to you if you were a newborn or even what would it feel like as a human being? For example, what does it feel like to you when you are in a dark place to emerge with a bright light in your eyes? If someone were to surprise you with a large object jabbed into your mouth, what would it feel like? Take into consideration lighting, noise, sensations and support. Do you want your baby's first experience to be infused by chemical opiates and medication?

Once upon a time, they used to smack a baby when it emerged from its mother. Today, they know this practice creates shock and psychological damage in the infant. In many places in North America they are ending the practice of routine suctioning of the baby, since it is associated with mouth trauma and can lead to the baby experiencing difficulties when breastfeeding. There are more and more practices that are being eliminated because of the harm they do to the baby.

Ultimately, it is your body and your baby, so the decision is yours alone to make. The key is to research all the options and risks for both you and your baby and follow your inner guidance.

Develop a Pregnancy Plan

Plans are of little importance, but planning is essential.

~ Winston Churchill

Establish your most important prenatal priorities. What are the most important things you can do for your self while pregnant? What are the most important things you can do for your baby? What are the most important things you can do for your relationship with your partner?

Planning is a wonderful way to help alleviate stress. You can design a pregnancy plan to help create balance and prevent stress. Remember, plans don't always go exactly the way that you want them to go so make sure that you allow room for movement in your plan.

When you create a pregnancy plan, break it down into the trimesters. Review and update your plan when you move into a new trimester to make sure that the plan continues to meet your needs. It is also a good idea to follow a prenatal book week-by-week so you can make changes to your plan as you progress through your pregnancy. These are some helpful questions for you to consider:

- *When will I tell my family and friends that I'm pregnant?*

- *When will I take maternity leave?*

- *When will I let work know?*

- *How am I going to relax?* Make sure that you list nourishing relaxation strategies and fun activities in your pregnancy plan.

- *What ways will I stay healthy during my pregnancy?* Plan out your rest and exercise strategies, nutritional needs, meals and ways that you will unwind. Allow your baby to be your inspiration for staying healthy during this time.

- *What ways can I develop a deepening intimacy with my partner?* Plan weekly dates and daily activities you can do with your partner.

Develop a Birthing Plan

I always say don't make plans, make options.

~Jennifer Aniston

In addition to your pregnancy plan, it is important to have a birth plan ready to clarify your needs and preferences for your baby's birthday. One of the best resources available on birthing options is a book titled *Pregnancy, Childbirth and the Newborn: The Complete Guide* by Penny Simkin et al. I have included an overview of what you could include into your birth plan:

Education. The first step is to educate yourself on the birthing options available to you and your partner. A doula is a great resource to learn about your options. You can also read books or watch movies that share positive birthing information in detail. It is important to decide your preferences and share them with your doula, midwife or obstetrician long before your due date. Bring a copy of your birth plan with you to your birthing facility. Participate in all decisions to ensure that you and your baby's needs are met.

The Team - Who will be your professional support team to assist you in the birth of your baby: midwife, obstetrician, general physician and/or doula?

The Location - Do you want to birth your baby at the hospital or would you be more comfortable at home or at a birthing center? Choose the most comfortable place for you.

People in the Room - You can have the option of having just you and your partner or you can bring in other family members and prenatal support. Choose only those who love and support you. If you are not at home, make sure that you let the facility know who is allowed in the room. You also have a say about whether or not you will allow medical or nursing students to be involved in your care. If you have a doula, inform the staff that you have one attending you. Also, be aware of any room limits in hospitals. Some only allow two or three visitors in the room at a time.

Room Setup - Before your due date, make sure that you go on the tour of the facility to make sure it is a good fit. Ask what birthing equipment is available:

birthing balls, birthing chairs, birth bar, birthing tub, a shower, etc. Find out what options are readily available, which ones you will need to bring in yourself and what you will need to book for your big day. If you are birthing at home, plan what you will need and which room(s) you will choose for birthing.

Plan What You Will Bring - Find out what you can bring to the birthing location. Can you bring in food from your home or do you need to eat from their menu? Will they allow you to eat? You may want to bring basic items like your birth plan, toiletries, money for parking, an oversized delivery shirt, a sarong, departure clothing, breastfeeding (bra) pads, massage oil and reading material. For the baby, you may need a car seat, a blanket, an outfit and diapers. Other items may include music, a special pillow or a comfy blanket.

Atmosphere - Whether at home or at a facility, a positive environment in the room helps alleviate stress during childbirth. Possibilities include low lighting, music and privacy. As a birthing women's sense of smell can be extremely heightened, scented items can often be annoying and uncomfortable. Ask people to refrain from wearing perfume or scented products.

Logistics - Make a list of all the practical logistics you'll need to prepare for the big day: how you'll get there, the route you'll take, where you need to check in, drop off strategies, if cafeteria/food is available for visitors, whether parking is available and the cost of parking.

Induction Options - Although this may not always be an option, you can make some decision on how you will be induced, if it is necessary. Will your membranes be broken artificially? Do you want the doctor to administer medications to induce childbirth? Do you want to use natural methods such as moxibustion or acupressure? Be clear on what your first preferences are for induction and then only use the other alternatives if needed. If there is no medical reason, consider giving your baby a little more time to develop within you. The risks associated with induction of labor include increased risk of premature birth, instrumental interventions,[64] abnormal fetal heart rate, respiratory distress,[65] your baby being admitted to the neonatal intensive care unit,[66] delayed breastfeeding and cesarean surgery.[67]

Pain Management - Determine how you would like to manage the pain. Decide whether you'll have an IV narcotic, an epidural analgesia or natural birth. Whatever you decide make sure that you remain flexible during the process, you may change your mind. If the birth will be medicated, discuss the options with your health care provider. Ask about side effects for birthing and for the health of your baby. Remember that anything you are given, your baby also receives. If a side effect is nausea for you, just think about what your baby may be also experiencing. Drugs affect your baby's experience of childbirth and can even affect your newborns mental and physical development.

If you choose a natural birth, what breathing and pain relief strategies can you learn ahead of time to help ease childbirth? Will you use water submersion as an effective way to prevent or relieve pain? Have you considered Lamaze, the Bradley Method or Hypnobirthing techniques?

Positions and Techniques for Comfort - Certain medications and monitoring may prevent you from moving and utilizing effective birthing positions. If you have had an epidural or are attached to a monitor you may still have the option of moving into a variety of positions such as side-lying, semi-prone, semi-sitting, supported squat and classical knees into the chest.

For women who choose natural birthing, there are numerous positions and techniques available to speed labor and ease pain during childbirth including standing, swaying, walking, slow dancing, squatting, leaning forward with support while standing or sitting, sitting upright, rocking in a chair, open knee position while lying forward, standing lunge, side-lying, being on all fours and many more. Changing positions can also help if a baby is not descending or is malpositioned.

The Level of Monitoring - You can decide on the amount of monitoring that you would like: continuous, intermittent or no monitoring. Generally, the more monitoring that you get, the less mobility you will have during childbirth. In addition, continuous monitoring is associated with an increase in instrumental vaginal births and cesarean surgeries.[68]

Even though intermittent auscultation of fetal heart rate is an accepted practice in low risk labors in many countries, hospitals in the US have disregarded recommendations against continuous monitoring for low risk women.[69] Continuous monitoring is required for high-risk conditions. If continuous monitoring is required do not spend your time watching the monitor. Focus internally instead.

One additional type of monitoring is internal fetal heart rate monitoring. Internal monitoring requires your bag of waters to be broken and a wire electrode to be attached to the scalp of the baby. Recent research indicates that internal monitoring does not significantly reduce the rate of cesarean surgeries, nor does it decrease the number of adverse neonatal outcomes.[70] If you are having a low risk birth, consider opting out of internal fetal monitoring.

Newborn Baby Care - If you give birth in a hospital, there are many routine procedures that hospitals automatically perform that may not be in the best interest of your baby. As a parent, you get to decide whether or not any procedures are performed, but it is important that you inform the staff ahead of time. In addition, it is important that you assign either your partner or a guardian to ensure your wishes are honored, as you will need to rest and may not be able to express your wishes after birthing. To get a full list of procedures, either contact your health care provider or the hospital ahead of time.

- **Holding Your Baby** – First and foremost, make it known to everyone assisting you that you want to immediately hold your baby skin to skin. Communicate that any procedure, if any, will be done in your arms or by your side.

- **Suctioning** – Suctioning has been linked to mouth injuries, emotional trauma and an aversion to breastfeeding. Only 5-10% of newborns require active resuscitation. As long as the cord has not been clamped or injured, and the cord is still pulsing, the baby receives oxygen from the placenta. You can request that suctioning be done only if an emergency arises. Hospitals have begun to eliminate routine suctioning, but voice your preferences to ensure that it is not done unnecessarily.

- **Cord Clamping** – There are many advantages to your baby's health when you delay the clamping of the cord. One of the most important is that your baby continues to receive vital oxygen and nutrients so your baby's system can transition naturally to begin the process of breathing from its lungs. The benefits of delayed cord clamping also include improved oxygenation of the brain in the first 24 hours[71] and protection from intraventricular hemorrhage and late-onset sepsis.[72] Just delaying the clamping of the umbilical cord for two minutes decreases the need for transfusion[73] and increases iron stores by 27 to 47 mg.[74] Early clamping is harmful to the newborn, as it denies them additional blood supply. The side effects of premature cord clamping include decreased access to additional blood supply, higher incidences of hemorrhaging, anemia (low iron), decreased tissue oxygenation and increased need for ventilation. Note: If you have chosen to extract cord blood for stem cell storage, you are required to clamp the cord early. One disadvantage to extracting cord blood is that your baby is denied immediate use of necessary stem cells at birth and may actually increase the likelihood of childhood disease.

- **Cord Cutting –** The advantages of delaying cord cutting are synonymous with delaying cord clamping. Unless there is a medical emergency, there are no physical benefits to cutting the cord early.

- **PKU Test –** A phenylketonuria test is administered to ensure a newborn has the enzyme required to use phenylalanine. If the enzyme is not present, a baby risks brain damage. The method entails poking the newborn's heel to collect a blood sample. The test needs to be done 24 hours after birth and within a few days from birth. Make sure they warm the heel of your baby first. If the test is done earlier, it may be inaccurate.

- **Silver Nitrate or Antibiotic Eye Ointment –** This procedure is performed to prevent blindness from exposure to maternal gonorrhea during childbirth. Ensure you get screened for sexually transmitted infections (STIs) long before your due date. If you have had a recent STI test and your test confirms you don't have an infection, opt out of the procedure. However, some states mandate this practice regardless of whether a baby is born vaginally or by cesarean. The side effects of administration can include clogged tear ducts, redness, swelling and blurred vision.

- **Vitamin K Injection** – Unless you direct the staff otherwise, a Vitamin K injection will most likely be given to your baby within six hours after birth. Since the psychological effects of intramuscular injections of newborns are unknown, you may want to request an oral dose instead to prevent unnecessary stress on your baby. Discuss this option with your midwife or obstetrician ahead of time, as it may require you to pick up a prescription prior to the birth. Vitamin K is administered to enhance blood clotting and to prevent hemorrhagic disease of the newborn. It is also required for high-risk babies who are born preterm, have liver challenges, have experienced breathing difficulties or bruising during birth, are born by caesarean section, forceps or vacuum or whose mothers have taken drugs for epilepsy or tuberculosis during pregnancy.

- **Hepatitis B Vaccine** – This vaccine is given to prevent the risk of Hep B in newborns with parents who are intravenous drug users, diagnosed with STIs, tattoo and body piercing recipients, health care workers and at high risk for contracting Hep B. While pregnant, get tested for Hep B to determine if you have been infected. If you are free of Hep B, and your state allows it, consider opting your newborn out of this vaccination or delaying it until your baby is older. It is interesting to note that Canada does not perform routine Hep B vaccinations on newborns.

- **Bathing** – Your baby's skin will be extremely sensitive to touch and temperature after birthing. Sensory overload from washcloths and cleansers can feel overwhelming. Vernix, the coating on your baby's skin, is there for a specific purpose. It moisturizes and protects your baby from infection. Consider opting out of or delaying a bath entirely. Instead, you can gently massage the vernix into your baby's skin.

- **Circumcision** – I recognize this is a personal and often cultural issue. Please note that the American Academy of Pediatrics (AAP) does not support circumcision, as there are no proven medical benefits to the procedure. There are significant side effects and risks to circumcision, which include pain and stress, sleep disruption, interference with breastfeeding, curvature of the penis, Fournier's syndrome, erectile dysfunction, infection, interference with breastfeeding, intolerance to pain for six months after surgery, staphylococcal scalded skin syndrome, psychological trauma and orgasm difficulties.[75] [76]

Emergencies - Lastly, write down what you would like to see happen in the event of an emergency. If an unexpected cesarean is necessary, your original birthing plan will need a contingency plan so you still have some influence over what is happening.

- Let your health care professional know if you would like to be awake for the surgery.
- Would you like your partner to attend to you or the baby?
- Would you like to see and hold the baby before they run tests?
- Would you like music playing in the surgery room?
- Are you comfortable with the surgical staff chatting during your surgery?

Remember that this is your birth so make sure that it has everything that is important to you. Prepare your birth plan with the preferences for your birthing experience and give a copy to the health care professionals who will be assisting the birth. Just like a pregnancy plan, allow room for changes since some deliveries may not go according to plan.

Include Your Partner in Any Pregnancy Planning

Your husband may not be a wealth of pregnancy information,
but he is a wealth of 'you' information.

~Erin MacPherson, The Christian
Mama's Guide to Having a Baby

Make your pregnancy a partnership. Involving your partner in the planning of your pregnancy and childbirth is beneficial to you, your partner and your baby. Begin discussions early and find time to plan.

With pregnancy planning, discussing what your needs are and hearing your partner's needs is an important part of each of you feeling supported during your pregnancy and helps to strengthen your bond with your partner. When you feel supported, life feels less stressful and the baby has the benefit of having a more peaceful prenatal experience.

In addition, your partner feels like an important part of the experience. Not only is this beneficial for the two of you, but it also gives your partner the opportunity to more fully bond with the baby.

When you discuss your pregnancy plan with your partner, keep an open mind. Suggest that both of you read all of the same books and share your reflections on the content with each other. As you both become educated, begin to write down the strategies and experiences you'd both like to experience. Remember to consider what your baby would like, as well.

Always take the time to schedule pregnancy and birth planning sessions and be sure to review them several times during the pregnancy, as your partner may want to become even more active as you get closer to the due date. Attend as many prenatal appointments together as you can to ensure your partner feels included and informed.

Keys to effective pregnancy and birthing planning with your partner:
- Communicate your needs.
- Discover your partner's needs.
- Establish a format where you can share with each other.
- Understand your partner's limitations and patterns.
- Come up with a vision of how you'd like to experience your relationship while pregnant.
- Express gratitude and appreciation.

Create a Pregnancy Budget

Any sensible family has a budget that lays out how much will be spent for household and other purposes. Without such planning, things would quickly go awry.

~ Walter Ulbricht

Having a baby can be a very expensive endeavor. Although you will have ongoing expenses when your baby arrives, there are a number of expenses that you can be faced with before baby arrives. For this reason, it is important

118

to create a pregnancy budget that reflects what you will need to spend to get ready for the baby and for at least a year after the birth. Also, remember to factor in any changes to your income you may experience once your baby is born.

Creating a pregnancy budget is actually quite simple, but it does mean that you really need to be honest with yourself about your budget. Baby items cost a lot of money and if you have a very small budget, you will need to look for less expensive items, purchase used items or receive previously used items from friends. To save money, limit the number of outfits in each phase of growth for the baby, as you will discover that s/he grows quickly into new sizes.

In addition, don't feed into the 'must haves' that magazines and advertisers influence you to buy. Although there are a thousand different things you can purchase, you will probably only really use a dozen of them in the long run. Ask other parents what they couldn't live without and what items they found to be a waste of money.

Medical bills and costs for extended prenatal support should also be factored in. If you have health care coverage, then this isn't a big worry but you should remember that some things are not covered. If you don't have health care, then be prepared for the expense of birthing your baby. If you have private insurance that covers birthing expenses, be prepared to cover the cost of a significant deductible.

Once you have a list, look at your own wants and needs and give them a priority. For example, a high chair isn't necessary until baby is sitting upright, so it can wait until later to be purchased. Put it in your budget, as a purchase with low priority.

Once you know what items you'd like to purchase and have figured out how much everything costs, determine how much money you will put aside each month to start saving for what you need.

Sort Out Your Finances

A big part of financial freedom is having your heart
and mind free from worry about the what-ifs of life.

~ *Suze Orman*

Sorting out your finances goes hand in hand with creating a pregnancy budget and will help you alleviate a large chunk of your stress. In fact, many people can equate the majority of their stress to monetary problems so it is important to get your finances under control.

- **Determine where you stand.** To sort out your finances, start collecting all of your bills, list your monthly expenses, and figure out what outstanding debts you owe.

- **Consolidate your debt.** Debt consolidation entails taking out one loan to pay off many others. The benefit is that you may be able to secure a lower interest rate. Make sure your payments can fit into your budget or it will just cause unnecessary stress. Consolidating debt makes it easier to deal with one payment per month and eliminates calls from creditors.

- **Consider bankruptcy.** If your debt has become unmanageable, definitely consider filing for bankruptcy. Contact a credit counselor or search online for bankruptcy advice. There are pros and cons to bankruptcy, so do your research and make sure you receive services from an approved credit counselor.

- **Make a budget and stick to it.** Make sure that you are not spending more than you make and put a portion of your earnings into a savings account you cannot touch. Separate needs from wants. Sticking to a budget will quickly get your finances in order and will greatly reduce your stress. There are books available that go into detail on how to effectively budget.

- **Eliminate debt.** If possible, pay off all your debt. Once your debt is paid, set up healthy financial habits to ensure you never incur debt again.

- **Ask for help.** If your family is struggling financially, assistance may be available from family members, friends or programs in the area you live. Begin with asking for assistance on how to improve your financial situation rather than asking to be rescued.

- **Apply for financial aid.** If you use a hospital for your birth, consider applying for financial assistance programs for the medical expenses or try negotiating with the hospital to significantly reduce your hospital bills.

- **Breath.** Take a deep breath in through your nose and let it out through your mouth. Use EFT (review the section called "Use Emotional Freedom Technique") to release financial stress from your body with statements such as, "Even though I feel stressed about my finances, I fully and completely love and accept myself."

Simplify Your Space & Get Organized

Simplicity is the ultimate sophistication.

~ Leonardo da Vinci

Living and working in an organized, clutter free and clean space is a great way to experience a peaceful state of mind. Think of how you feel when you walk into a home that is clean and clutter free versus a home that is dirty and disorganized.

Removing clutter can seem like an impossible task if you don't know where or how to start. Simply get rid of or donate anything you do not use. Stop collecting. Clear off your shelves and countertops. Establish a place for every item, whether it is in a drawer, filing system, closet or shelf. I find that by having a place for everything, my house remains uncluttered. Stop buying unnecessary things. Use a strategy where you get rid of an item every time you purchase another item. For example, if you buy a shirt donate an old shirt to a charity organization. If you are on the fence with some items, create a 'maybe box' that you can store out of the way. Check on it in six months to see if you've used it.

Get rid of any clothes that no longer fit you. Donate, gift or sell most of your books except your favorites. And finally, donate or recycle your old newspapers and magazines.

Simplify and de-clutter. Have a box for unwanted items and as you organize an area, toss anything you no longer use or want. Or schedule a day where you and your partner gather unwanted items from every area of the house and donate them or have a garage sale.

122

If a drawer or closet is overflowing with items, get rid of some of them or find another area that they can reside in. I've been in homes where they have 500 plastic shopping bags bursting out of a drawer or from under the kitchen sink. I coach people to let go of the need to hang on to everything.

What areas need the most organizing? Begin one step at a time. Every week, I pick one dresser or a closet to de-clutter. That way I don't feel overwhelmed. If I have more time that day then I tackle another area. If you have a designated junk drawer, clean it out once a month. You'd be surprised at how good it feels. Getting organized is a great way to reduce stress, especially for an expecting mom. Organizing is an activity that pregnant women feel helps them prepare their home for the arrival of their baby.

While organizing, make sure the fun and nostalgic items you find don't distract you from your task. Instead, set them aside to enjoy when your task is complete.

Need additional support?
- Hire a professional organizer to assist you.
- Get your partner involved by assigning areas for your partner to organize. Remember to assign the tasks in chunks so their whole day isn't taken up with a task. People tend to be better at organizing areas they are familiar with, so have them organize their own dresser or closet. Your partner may be better suited for organizing the garage, attic or hard to reach areas while you are pregnant.

Create a Clean Space

We adore chaos because we love to produce order.

~ M. C. Escher

Every Sunday, my husband and I take two hours to organize and clean using a step-by-step system I'll call the **Fast Cleaning System.** We are fairly efficient and know both what needs to be accomplished and our specific roles in getting things done. It makes a great difference in our state of mind for the week to have an organized house. The added benefit is that I am not left doing all of the work by myself.

It wasn't always easy. In the beginning of our relationship, I noticed I was the one doing the majority of cleaning. My husband shared he didn't see what needed to be done in the way I could. He recommended that I tell him exactly what needed to be done, because he couldn't figure it out. I organized and implemented a cleaning system by directing him step by step. He eventually learned the system and some Sundays he starts without me. Overall, I find most people thrive when you give them defined tasks with expected outcomes and celebrate their participation.

A benefit to using this system is that when guests are coming over for special visits or your parents are coming for an impromptu visit, you have a quick strategy for cleaning.

If you implement a system like this with your partner, I recommend you print off a version of this list that divides up the household tasks evenly so that your partner can get a visual of the organizing and cleaning road map.

Ground Rules:

- Set a schedule.

- Make it fun. Put on some upbeat music that you both enjoy to inspire a swift implementation of organization and cleaning.

- Convey your standards. Most, but not all, guys have a strategy of doing the very minimum when cleaning. I have a simple motto: "If it isn't clean, then it isn't clean, so do it again." With men, this simply happens because one or more possibilities: vision problems, low standards/not caring, not knowing how to clean something properly, not enough attention to detail and trying to get you to do it.

- Stick to your assigned tasks. The "trying to get you to do it" strategy is a favorite strategy that many men learn at a young age with their mothers. Too many women get frustrated with low cleaning standards and throw in the towel and decide to clean things instead of getting guys to do it. Be firm; do not do your partner's assigned tasks for them. If they don't do a great job, send them back until it is clean.

- Don't get caught up in organizing the micro. Avoid sorting through drawers or going through papers. This can be done at another time or once the overall clean is completed. When people get caught up in going through things, it slows down the process.

- Assign a place for every item. Part of staying organized is creating a consistent place for everything. Every book, piece of paper, article of clothing, dish, trinket and tool needs to have somewhere it normally resides when not in use. The benefit is that it can be found by anyone who is looking for it and it is easy to put away. If you don't have a place for something, then create one. Get a few plastic, bamboo or cardboard containers or boxes to keep smaller items in and label them. Organize like items with similar items.

- Have a goal to keep furniture and counters free of items.

Fast Cleaning System

Before cleaning any one room. We start with a simple strategy of moving all items to the rooms they normally reside in when not in use. Here are the steps we use:

1. Gather all dirty laundry to be washed. Have everyone bring their own laundry to a central place and grab what needs to be cleaned from the bathrooms and kitchen. Start a load of laundry.

2. Set out a garbage can and a recycle bin.

3. Then starting in the living room, and moving into other rooms, systematically collect and pile items according to the rooms they belong to and then take them to their rooms. Once in another room do the same thing until all rogue items are in their rightful rooms. Do not immediately put things away; just leave the items for now. Collect all paper and items to be recycled and place them in the recycle bin as you go from room to room.

4. Now begin to clean room by room. Have one person clean the whole kitchen while the other cleans the whole bathroom. If you have more than one bathroom, then you can split up the bathrooms or have one person do them all. In each room, start by clearing off anything that

is on the floors. Then clear off all surfaces such as countertops, the tops of furniture and shelves.

5. One person vacuums the whole house while the other dusts with a damp rag.

6. Assign each of you one drawer or closet per week to organize. Take out everything, clean it, toss out or donate what you don't need.

7. File all papers into a filing system.

8. Collect and take garbage out to garbage cans.

9. Celebrate with a high five, a hug and a kiss!

Make a List

In all planning you make a list and you set priorities.

~Alan Lakein

Many financially successful and famous people use lists to keep them focused and on track. Making lists decreases stress, clears your mind, helps you to become more organized and allows you to manage your time effectively. On the other hand, avoid creating a list that is too long, as it will lead to overwhelm and stress. Be realistic about what you can accomplish in your time frame and refrain from pushing yourself to accomplish too much at one time. It is important to use your lists to create structure in your day, however remain flexible when you can't accomplish everything.

The key to creating lists is making sure you prioritize the most important tasks to complete and schedule time to complete your lists. You can also identify the items on your list that can be delegated to others, which can help reduce your workload and stress. I have a list for my husband that he can check when he has spare time on the weekends. I also create a fun list of unique activities we can do together as a couple, which are inspired by articles on local companies, restaurant reviews or event postings.

Other helpful lists include: a to do list, a grocery list, a list of goals, a dream list of things you'd like to experience in this lifetime and a personal pleasure list of activities that make you smile and reduce stress.

You can even create a prenatal list of things you'd like to accomplish before the baby arrives. The list can include items to buy, classes to take, foods to eat, topics to discuss with your partner and preferred baby names.

Read a Good Book

Books are the quietest and most constant of friends; they are the most accessible and wisest of counselors, and the most patient of teachers.

~ Charles W. Eliot

If you love to read, you don't need to hear from me about the value of a great fictional story or fascinating autobiography. However, if it has been a while since you've enjoyed a book, find one that appeals to you and just dive in. You'd be surprised at how many books out there are emotionally moving, deeply interesting, creative or profoundly inspiring.

Reading Can Reduce Stress

There is something about reading that is simultaneously relaxing and mentally stimulating at the same time. The imagination and creativity of the mind becomes activated. An independent study in the UK found that reading reduces stress levels by 68% and that it only takes six minutes of silent reading to slow the heart rate and ease muscle tension.[77] The findings also revealed that reading was more effective at reducing stress than listening to music, going for a walk or sitting down with a cup of tea.

An alternative to reading a book is to lie down, relax, close your eyes and listen to an audio version. My husband loves to listen to books while on vacation or doing chores around the house. On nights I've had trouble falling asleep, I've dosed off quickly while listening to a chapter of an audio book.

Educate Yourself With Prenatal Books

I have never known any distress that an
hour's reading did not relieve.

~ Charles de Montesquieu

Prenatal books are brilliant tools to learn more about the pregnancy journey and the birthing process. Pregnancy and birthing books, by authors like Penny Simkin and Ina May Gaskin, are great starting points for reducing stress and anxiety around childbirth and empowering you.

With the wide range of prenatal books available, I recommend that parents find books that fit their lifestyle and address their needs. Prenatal books cover just about everything you will ever need to know and they are an invaluable resource to boosting your confidence as an expecting mom.

Here are some examples of the content prenatal books offer:

- *Break down of development.* Knowing how your baby is growing is very important.

- *Advice for parents.* Although most books offer plenty of advice for a new mom, it is important to find a book that offers advice for your partner to address additional concerns and questions.

- *Prenatal nutrition.* It is important to know what foods are best for you and your baby during pregnancy and while breastfeeding.

- *Birth planning.* Look for books that give you tips, options and advice on planning for the birth of your baby. Having a clear birth plan will help reduce prenatal stress.

- *Shared experiences.* Hearing positive pregnancy and birthing stories assists expecting moms to feel safe in their own birthing experience.

I recommend that you avoid reading about prenatal or birthing complications. While it is important to be aware of risks, focusing or worrying about the risks can often bring about the very situation women want to avoid. Instead focus on books and information that inspire healthful strategies for pregnancy, birthing and breastfeeding. See appendix for recommended reading resources.

Lastly, take the time to find some wonderful children's books for your baby. Some old classics or new favorites can be read to your baby while you are pregnant and will encourage your child's development, aid in bonding and put you in a state of relaxation.

Have Fun & Laugh

A smile starts on the lips, a grin spreads to the eyes, a chuckle comes from the belly; but a good laugh bursts forth from the soul, overflows, and bubbles all around.

~ *Carolyn Birmingham*

Laughter is amazing and is a simple key to happiness and health. If you've ever found yourself unable to stop laughing, uncontrollable laughter can be one of those experiences that remain etched in your mind. I remember a time I couldn't stop laughing when I was seven years old. I don't even remember what it was about, but I can remember the cramping in my stomach and yet that seemed to make me laugh more!

I also attended laughter yoga a few times and remember taking my sister with me. The two of us could not stop laughing. It is a memory I will never forget. What joy! I've had many experiences of laughing throughout my life that I can touch into and recall, all anchored in my cellular memory with laughter.

In addition to anchoring fantastic memories, laughter is one of the cheapest and easiest forms to relieve stress in the body and mind. Gelatology (the study of laughter) documents the myriad of physical, mental and emotional health benefits of laughing. Some of the awesome benefits of laughter include:

- Decreased stress hormones
- Reduction of pain
- Improved mood
- Relaxation of the body and mind
- Reduced mental stress

- Increased memory and learning
- Increased production of antibodies and helper T-cells that are vital to fighting and preventing disease[78]
- Stabilization of blood pressure
- Improved digestion
- Increased lung ventilation
- Strengthening the immune system
- Increased endorphins
- Protection of the heart[79]
- Assisting us to bond with others
- Oxygenates the blood

Laughter during pregnancy benefits both the mother and the baby because we know that if mom is healthier, baby is healthier.

Ways to Create Opportunity for Laughter
- Cultivate friendships with humorous people.
- Spend time with fun people or happy children.
- Join a laughter club or go to a laughter yoga class.
- Make a toddler laugh and you'll be laughing along.
- Go to YouTube and listen to videos of babies and children laughing; the joy is infectious!
- Bring humor into conversations.
- Watch a comedy.
- Find time to be playful and silly.

Smile

Every time you smile at someone, it is an action of love,
a gift to that person, a beautiful thing.

~ Mother Teresa

I love to see people smile! As a universal symbol of happiness, a smile is uplifting and positively infectious. People who smile are perceived more positive, kind, honest and funny. Research studies have shown that smiling makes you happy. By producing facial expressions, such as smiling, you can create similar biochemical effects on the body, as those that result from actual emotions, such as happiness.[80]

One research study reported that by making the "e" sound, which mimics the facial characteristics of a smile, that subjects reported feeling good. It was found that facial changes involved in smiling have direct effects on certain brain activities associated with happiness.[81]

One of the practices I recommend is smiling to your baby in your belly. It is a simple way to improve your mood and to bond with your baby. You can also extend this action to any part of your body such as your heart centre, liver, intestines, brain or skin. For an additional boost, go for a walk and smile to a tree, the ocean, the planet or the universe!

Connect With Your Baby

I think it is such a privilege to give a baby its first home inside your body. [After the pregnancy was over] I found myself massaging my stomach gently. I miss him being in my body -- stretching, hiccupping even. It was a wonderful, deep, loving, fulfilling feeling.

~ Celine Dion

Remember you and your baby are one. Talking, singing, reading and acknowledging your baby are great ways to connect and bond. Research shows that prenatal bonding strengthens your connection after your baby is born and assists in your baby's physical and emotional development.

Although the auditory perception and learning for fetuses begins in the third trimester, as soon as you conceive you can begin communicating non-verbally or verbally to your baby through reading, writing, singing or talking. Express your gratitude and love to your baby and be mindful of what you say or feel. Your baby also experiences the emotional states you experience.

Gently caress your baby through your belly. The loving touch is registered by your body biochemically through oxytocin and other stress reducing hormones. Your baby is then bathed in oxytocin and love. If things are not going well, let your baby know that you are having a challenging day and that you love him/her anyway.

Not only is it important to bond prenatally with your baby, it is also important to encourage intimacy between you and your partner, as the release of oxytocin in love making and touching assists you in bonding with your baby. Researchers have found that high levels of oxytocin[82] in the first trimester and across pregnancy were closely related to how maternal mothers would be after the birth of their baby and how connected they would feel.

At about the 26th to 28th week, if you haven't started already, this is a great time to begin to sing, read or speak out loud to your baby. Studies have shown that fetuses recognize and respond to their mother's voice over a female stranger's voice when played outside the body.[83] There is also evidence that the fetus can access the mother's speech through bone conduction.[84] When you communicate verbally to your baby it contributes to your baby's brain development, physical development, communication skills and hearing skills.

By the time of birth, your baby responds to the language you've been speaking over unfamiliar languages, demonstrating the ability for a fetus to learn the properties of language such as pitch, some aspects of rhythm and some phonetic information.[85] Researchers have also demonstrated that fetuses have long-term memory in relationship to melodic sound.[86]

Fetuses receive sound of more than 40 decibels, so avoid putting speakers against your belly as it can over stimulate the developing auditory system or may interfere with your baby's sleep/wake cycle. Normal conversation is approximately 60 dBs, a refrigerator is 40 dBs and a vacuum cleaner is 80 dBs.

Take a Relaxing Bath With
Magnesium Bath Salts

Magnesium is indeed the unsung hero and is a key nutraceutical
that everybody needs to know about.

~ Dr. Stephen T. Sinatra

Mmmm, bathing in water feels beautifully relaxing and refreshing. I imagine the therapeutic benefits of bathing in water have been known from the beginning of human existence. There are many references in religious and historical texts, stories and mythologies that share the uses and benefits of water, as well as the sacredness of water. In many areas of the world today, bathing in water is considered an extreme luxury and a sacred privilege.

Over the years, bathing in water has been a stress reliever for me. Taking baths is great way to unwind after a very difficult day as it has a relaxing and beneficial effect on the body and mind. While pregnant, the buoyancy of water has been known to help relieve pressures, aches and pains associated with accommodating a growing baby.

In addition to the many benefits of bathing in water, adding magnesium salts to your bath can be a great opportunity to absorb some magnesium into the body and to draw out toxins from the body. Very few people realize the importance of magnesium to muscle and nerve functions, normal brain functioning and intestinal health. Among US adults, it is suggested that at least 68% of the population is deficient in magnesium.[87]

Magnesium is essential for calcium absorption and bone health. Without it the body cannot utilize the calcium in your diet. Magnesium also works with calcium to assist with blood clotting and regulating blood pressure. In addition, magnesium and calcium work to improve health functioning of the lungs, the immune system and energy metabolism. Research suggests that patients with acute migraines register with low levels of ionized magnesium.[88] Stress, poor nutrition and genetic inability to absorb magnesium are some of the reasons why migraine sufferers may be lacking in magnesium.

Magnesium deficiency has also been associated with ADD, ADHD, Alzheimer's, arrhythmias, asthma, cancers, calcium deficiency, Crohn's disease, depression, diabetes, eczema, hair loss, heart attacks, insomnia, muscle wasting, nail fungus, osteoporosis, PMS, psoriasis, tooth decay, Tourette's syndrome, twitches and many more chronic and autoimmune diseases.

During pregnancy, women who are deficient in magnesium may also show symptoms such as leg cramps, pre-eclampsia, toxemia of pregnancy, fluid retention and restless legs.

A great way to access magnesium is in the magnesium rich foods we eat, such as dark leafy greens, vegetable juices, molasses, soaked pumpkin seeds, soaked almonds, okra, dark chocolate and kombu kelp. However, the skin can also absorb magnesium from time spent in the ocean or in a bath that has added magnesium chloride bath salts.

Note: Magnesium sulfate is commonly known as Epsom salts. Although Epsom salts have a beneficial effect and can be used, they are not as effective as magnesium chloride bath salts or magnesium oil. Check your local natural food store or go online to see if a retailer sells magnesium oil or magnesium chloride bath salts in your area.

Bath Temperature

When bathing, try to keep your water temperature just above body temperature. A warm bath feels relaxing and invigorating. Although many people attempt to bathe in the hottest water they can withstand, very hot baths can create stress on the body by using up energy to try to cool itself down internally and baths that are too hot can cause unnecessary stress on your baby.

Cool baths or foot soaks are great if you are feeling overheated. If you don't have time for a cool soak, you can rinse your wrists under cool water. Another way to refresh the body is to use a cool wet cloth to wipe down the backs of your knees, the inside of your arm, your chest, forehead and the back of your neck.

Get Wet

If there is magic on this planet, it is contained in water.

~ Loran Eisely, The Immense Journey, 1957

Water is a healing salve and everything from listening to water to placing your feet in water can be a calming experience. It is water that helps us relax and it is something that I strongly recommend using while you are pregnant. Whether you are swimming, sitting in the tub or standing in a shower, water can help wash away your stress and will also leave you feeling refreshed.

Some great ways to experience water during your pregnancy include:

✓ **Exercising in the water.** During pregnancy, swimming or aquatic-aerobic classes offer the stress relieving and health benefits of aerobic exercise combined with the physical stress reduction benefits due to buoyancy. Choose pools that are low in chlorine or use sodium chloride instead of chlorine, as researchers suggest that during pregnancy, trihalomethanes (chemical by-products of chlorine found in the water and air of indoor swimming pools) may present a risk to the mother and fetus and may be linked to miscarriage and low birth weight.[89]

✓ **Relaxing in water.** You can enjoy a relaxing shower or bath.

✓ **Soak your feet in water.** When your feet and ankles are tired from a day of work or being on your feet, enjoy a relaxing footbath. Fill a basin large enough for your feet with warm water. Dissolve approximately three tablespoons of aluminum free baking soda into the warm water and soak your feet as long as you feel comfortable. Dry your feet with a towel and ask your sweetheart to massage your feet with a little coconut oil or foot cream before you put on a clean pair of socks.

• **Playing in water.** Enjoy going to your local pool, a lake, or the ocean for a little swim or floating in water. The buoyancy effect of water pushing you up as your weight pushes down is simply delightful.

• **Birthing in warm water.** A water birth is a great method of relieving pain and relaxing the mother during childbirth. Researchers have concluded that water births are associated with a significantly shorter first stage of birthing,[90] a considerably less stressful and less painful birthing process, less use of pain medication, less vaginal trauma and less maternal infection[91] If hygiene is considered, water births are considered safe for both mother and baby.[92]

Water is very safe for you and your baby but it is important to follow a few recommendations so that it remains safe and enjoyable.

1. **Have someone available to assist you out of the tub during your last trimester when getting in and out of the tub can be difficult.**

2. **Keep water at between 97 to 99°F (36 to 37.2°C).** Although a nice hot bath can relieve tense muscles, you should never have a bath that is over 100°F (37.7°C). The reason for this is because the hotter the bath, the hotter you become and when you overheat your heart rate increases. This means that less blood is getting to your baby and it can put stress on your baby.

3. **Avoid saunas and hot tubs.** For the same reason as keeping baths cooler, avoid soaking in a sauna or hot tub. Again, this will overheat you and you can run the risk of putting unnecessary stress on your child.

4. **Use non-slip shoes or sandals when walking on wet surfaces.** Use non-slip bath mats and bath decals.

5. **Avoid the use of chemically fragranced bath salts, bubble baths, shower gels and bath foams.** Most bubble baths carry health warnings alerting their users about the possibility of skin irritation and urinary tract infections. Bubble baths have also been known to cause external vaginal itching and dry skin. Even if you seem to be ok with a chemically perfumed product, your baby is highly sensitive to chemicals as it develops.

6. **Avoid counterindicative essential oils.** The National Association for Holistic Aromatherapy (NAHA) has recommended that women avoid most aromatherapy uses in the first three months of pregnancy.

They have also recommended to avoid the use of the following essential oils while pregnant: basil, birch, cedar, cinnamon, clove bud, cypress, fennel, hyssop, jasmine, juniper, lemongrass, marjoram, myrrh, parsley, pennyroyal, peppermint, rockrose, rosemary, sage and thyme.

Stay Hydrated With Water

By the time it grows to be a full term baby, about a trillion cell divisions will have taken place. Every time a cell gives rise to a daughter cell, 75 percent or more of its volume has to be filled with water. In short, growth depends on the availability of water.

~ F. Batmanghelidj, MD, author of Water for Health, for Healing, for Life

When pregnant, it is very important that you stay hydrated throughout your day. Your water needs increase as your pregnancy progresses because you are producing plasma, blood and amniotic fluid for development of the fetus. Since amniotic fluid replenishes itself approximately every hour, you need to adequately hydrate throughout your pregnancy. In addition, water can also help alleviate many side effects of pregnancy such as morning sickness, constipation, maternal overheating, water retention, leg cramps, joint pain and headaches.

Stress & Dehydration
When you are properly hydrated your brain, all other organs and the cells throughout your body operate efficiently and effectively. Research has shown that being dehydrated by two cups can create stress on your organs and can

increase your stress hormones. Dehydration during pregnancy can decrease fetal body and brain weight and can negatively affect fetal blood pressure.[93] In the third trimester, dehydration can also contribute to premature labor.

How Much Water?

Although it is a myth that you need to drink eight glasses of water a day, when you are pregnant, you may need to drink 8 or more glasses per day. Begin your day with a glass of water before you eat or drink anything else. Drink a glass of water 20 minutes prior to each major meal. This water provides the body with the hydration it needs to produce stomach acid for digesting your next meal.

Your additional water needs depend on your lifestyle. For example, if you eat water rich foods like fresh fruits and salads, you are receiving large quantities of water from your food. However, if you consume dry, dense, salted, spiced and processed foods, you will find you need to consume more water to help hydrate and flush the body. If you drink fresh vegetable juices, or other beverages, they can contribute to your hydration levels. Also, if you exercise or live in a hot climate, you will need to replenish any fluids you lose through sweating.

Learn to tune into your body periodically to check your hydration by assessing how your body and mind feel. If you feel hungry or thirsty, drink water. Your urine is also a great indicator of your levels of hydration. If it is very dark you need to drink more water. However, if it is very light, you may need to drink less.

Avoid sipping water throughout the day. On an empty stomach, sipping water delays the transfer of water from the stomach to the small intestine.

Have a glass or a few mouthfuls and move on.

Normally, the body is equipped to regulate and store water during sleep to keep itself hydrated. However, with increased water needs during pregnancy, you may find yourself thirsty in the middle of the night. If this occurs, drink at least a half a glass of water. Do your best to adequately hydrate during the day.

If you experience extreme thirst, consult with your health care provider.

Other Fluids

Although you can include other beverages into your daily fluid intake, it is important to drink pure water throughout your day. Fruit juice, milk, coffee and other processed liquids offer very little health benefits. Juice often contains a lot of sugar and other sweeteners that can add to unnecessarily high blood sugar levels for you and your baby. Caffeine can increase the risk of miscarriage and will also make you urinate more.

Researchers have determined that pasteurized milk subjects the organs, glands, bones and neurons to hormonal stimulation[94] and have found that the consumption of pasteurized cow milk is a linked to chronic diseases and symptoms typically found in Western societies, such as allergies, acne,[95] sinusitis,[96] post nasal drip, ear infections,[97] diabetes,[98] constipation,[99] anemia,[100] heart disease,[101] osteoporosis,[102] bloating and gas. Even worse, consuming milk while pregnant has been linked to developmental issues in fetuses, such as excessive birth weight.[103]

Commercial soymilk is highly over processed, contains synthetic (toxic) vitamin D and sweeteners. It has also been found to affect hormonal balance in the body due to excess phytoestrogens, potentially contributing to hypothyroidism[104] and premenopausal breast cancer.[105]

There really is no substitute for water when it comes to all of the benefits that it gives you. Not only does it help alleviate feelings of fatigue but it can also help you relax and reduces stress.

In addition, staying hydrated helps prevent water retention and alleviates pregnancy related swelling. It helps provide nutrients to your entire body and aids in sending those nutrients to your baby. Hydrating your body prevents bladder infections and helps prevent constipation. Drinking the right amount every day will ensure that your health is optimal and helps prevent health issues that could lead to chronic stress.

Not All Water is Beneficial

It is well known that most North American municipalities treat tap water with fluoride, chlorine dioxide, cleaners, disinfectants and even pharmaceuticals. While clean water is essential to maintaining a healthy body, research has also revealed that even small amounts of toxic chemicals such as chlorine or fluoride can affect not only long-term health, but also the health of future generations.

Drinking chlorinated tap water while pregnant may be linked to various birth defects and premature labor. Research studies have found that exposure to high levels of chlorination by-products may increase risks for fetal development issues such as cleft palate, neural development complications and heart defects.[106]

Regarding the fetus, fluoride is toxic to neural development. Researchers have found that in utero exposure to fluoride increases oxidative stress and causes imbalance on antioxidants, enzymes, proteins and cells in the central nervous system of the fetus.[107] Dental fluorosis is damage of dental enamel caused by excessive exposure to high concentrations of fluoride during tooth development of babies and children. Fluoride also interferes with proper thyroid functioning, resulting in interrupted DNA replication and repair, oxidative stress, decreased cell viability and induced cell death.[108] [109]

Fluoride in particular has been found to accumulate in high levels in the pineal gland and can lead to calcification of the gland. Calcification of the pineal gland is associated with insomnia, lumbar intervertebral disc degeneration, Alzheimer's disease, thickening of artery walls and aging. Researchers have noted that fluoride has been linked to accelerated sexual maturation in females[110] and is "likely to cause decreased melatonin production and to have other effects on normal pineal function, which in turn could contribute to a variety of effects in humans." [111]

Bottled water is often purified municipal water and is susceptible to dangerous toxins that could leach out of the plastic. Although great for removing some contaminants and chemicals, reverse osmosis water purification creates water that is devoid of minerals and is more acidic than most spring water.

Distilled water is free of bacteria, viruses and heavy metals. However, the water is fairly acidic and is mineral free. Distilled water is good for short-term detoxification. Carbon filtration systems are good for removing some organic chemical contaminants such as chlorine, pesticides and herbicides; however they do not eliminate most contaminants, nor do they influence pH and they are susceptible to mold.

Water ionizers produce ionized alkaline water through the process of electrolysis. Since alkaline water has a higher pH and an improved oxidation reduction potential (ORP) level than plain tap water, Japanese clinical studies suggest that it can neutralize acid in your bloodstream, improve your health, prevent disease, slow aging and boost your metabolism. However, these claims have yet to be verified by additional studies. There is one study out of Sweden that found pH extremes on either end to be problematic for human health.[112] Water ionizers are beneficial for short-term use. It is believed that long-term use can lead to health and digestive issues.

Optimal Water Choices

Make the best, most informed choice in your consumption of water for your health and the health of your baby. Whenever possible, drink mineral rich water from natural sources such as artesian or mountain spring water that is free of chlorine and sodium fluoride, has a pH close to 7, and is as vital and alive as possible. Research healthy water options in your area. In addition, eat organic, water rich, alkaline, living foods.

Stay Regular

Life is a tragedy of nutrition.

*~ Arnold Ehret, The Definite Cure
of Chronic Constipation*

Oh the ever so personal topic of pooping! I am just going to be candid, as I believe it serves to share experiences for educational purposes. I grew up with bowel movements that were infrequent and it wasn't until I met my husband that I realized the importance of averaging at least one bowel movement per day. He was surprised at how difficult and infrequently I passed my stool and suggested I go to the doctor. I didn't know any better, my parents never inquired, I never had conversations with my friends and the Internet didn't exist back then.

The doctor seemed just as ignorant as I was. She suggested that if I was regularly irregular than that was normal for me and to not worry about it. However, I knew something wasn't quite right in toilet land and so began my quest for intestinal health, which lead me to learning about all aspects of health and wellness.

Today, I celebrate bowel movements! Even among friends and with my sisters, I share when I've had a great "BM" with clapping and laughter. My sister finds this funny and has a giggle about it when I do my dance and she has been known to celebrate her victories with me, too. I do this to share with others the importance of not being ashamed and it sends a clear message to my body that it is a positive experience to let go of the waste and to not feel stressed about it.

The colon is very responsive to stress and can be affected when stress hormones are activated. Sources of stress can be emotional, physical, psychological or nutritional and they can result from current situations or early childhood experiences.

Importance of a Healthy Colon

In my research, I discovered how important intestinal health was to all areas of health in the body and mind. If you can learn to stay regular naturally, you'd be surprised at how everything else falls into place. When food digests too slowly, toxic by-products of digestion and fermentation can get absorbed into the body, contributing to disease, illness and unwanted weight gain. Feeling backed up and full of waste is uncomfortable, stressful and tiresome. When you experience regular and easeful bowel movements, you have more energy, feel lighter and freer.

An Ideal Bowel Movement

Healthy bowel movements occur 1-3 times every day, are soft, and leave the body with ease and without pain. If you experience constipation or abnormalities in your bowel movements, consult your health care provider. For long-term healthy intestinal solutions, eat well and reduce stress. If you are experiencing strain or discomfort, see the suggestions below to improve your digestion and evacuation.

- Pellet stool can be caused by stress, liver stagnation, lack of exercise, excessive red meat, wheat, sugar and alcohol.

- Soft, smelly stool may reveal that there is too much fat in your stool. This could be the result of too much fat in your diet, vitamin deficiency and bacterial overgrowth. If soft, smelly stool occurs regularly, it can indicate a medical condition of the intestines or pancreas.

- Chronic mucus in the stool may indicate inflammation in the intestines and is associated with intestinal conditions such as Crohn's disease, ulcerative colitis and celiac disease. Wheat allergies and sensitivities are very damaging to the colon and body (see the section "Eat a Balanced Diet" for information on wheat sensitivity). If it happens once in a blue moon, it is most likely associated with sensitivity to a food you've eaten. Mucus can also be present when you have a cold or flu.

Contributing Factors to Intestinal Health

Nutritional Stress

Diet plays an important role in maintaining a healthy colon. It is very difficult to get constipated if you eat a diet that is rich in raw, living plant foods, as these foods are high in minerals, vitamins, fiber and water. Processed foods that are low in fiber and high in poor quality fats contribute to constipation.

It is important to note, that it is not just the quantity of fiber, but also the quality of fiber that is important to intestinal health. There are many processed grocery items in boxes on market shelves that promote themselves as "high in fiber," but they are not healthy versions of fiber. Highly processed foods such as refined bran, wheat flour or any fortified foods are to be avoided. The healthiest fiber rich foods are fresh vegetables, greens and fruit, nuts, avocado and sprouted grains.

Eating large amounts of dairy and animal products can also contribute to constipation, as well as other health issues. See the section "Eat a Balanced Diet" for more tips on healthy nutritional choices.

Chewing

Digestion begins with the senses receiving the sights, smells and anticipation of food. Chewing functions to mechanically break down, moisten and infuse your food with the pre-digestion enzyme called amylase. It also activates the churning action in the stomach and small intestine.

Once amylase is released, it activates other enzymes to get ready for digestion. If you are interested in the proper digestion of your food, it is really important to chew your food until it is liquid. Most people do not adequately chew their food and the result is improperly digested food, which can lead to slow digestion, bloating, gas, constipation, acid reflux and strain on the pancreas. Over time, the strain on the pancreas can contribute to diabetes, adrenal fatigue, problems with the pituitary gland and then a cascade of other health issues.

Tips for Eating:

- Take small mouthfuls.
- Practice being mindful with your first bite.
- Chew your food until it is liquid.
- Do not wash food down with beverages or water.
- Chew your food with your mouth closed, breathing through the nose. Chewing with your mouth open or talking while eating can reduce the digestion of food and can result in taking in air with your food.
- Don't pick up more food until you have thoroughly chewed and swallowed your last bite.
- Avoid scraping your teeth with utensils.
- Avoid watching TV and movies while eating.
- Enjoy food with family and friends.

Dehydration

Our body needs water for every process and function it does, including the elimination of waste. Dehydration not only contributes to constipation, but also can create other symptoms in the body. The key to staying hydrated is to eat water rich foods (greens, fruit and vegetables) and drink fresh water.

Emotional Stress

I know far too many women who will not have a bowel movement with others in the same house or building. Some women absolutely will not go to the bathroom even with their partner in the house. While it is always much more relaxing to poop when you are alone, there is a gift in being able to have a bowel movement regardless of whom is around. The blessing is in honoring your body's need to evacuate waste.

Often stress around having bowel movements in the presence of others is related to early childhood events, where a person may have experienced stressful or negative feedback about toilet training, learned from another to fear public toilets or suffered embarrassment or shame around evacuation. Some of these issues can be buried deep into the subconscious because they are too painful to address or they could have occurred at a very young age. It may not be logical, but this kind of associated stress is automatic and intense.

As an adult, persistent negative emotions and emotional stress in the workplace, relationships or life in general can also trigger the activation of stress hormones, which can restrict or accelerate the movement of waste though the intestines.

One of the best techniques to clear stress around having bowel movements is to use EFT (review section entitled "Use Emotional Freedom Technique"). Try using any of these key phases that apply to your life:

- Even though I feel scared to have a bowel movement in a public place, I fully and completely love and accept myself.
- Even though I feel highly anxious to have a bowel movement when my partner is in the house, I fully and completely love and accept myself.

151

- Even though I feel stressed about having a bowel movement, I fully and completely love and accept myself.

- Even though my mom yelled at me when I was a child for not making it to the toilet, I fully and completely love and accept myself.

- Even though I feel stressed about work and I'm noticing I am backed up lately, I fully and completely love and accept myself.

- Even though I feel stressed about being pregnant and I find myself constipated, I fully and completely love and accept myself.

- Even though my hormones are affecting my bowel movements, I fully and completely love and accept myself.

Pregnancy

Once you are pregnant, hormonal influences can mildly affect the digestive tract by slowing gut transit. However, some women suffer from mild constipation prior to conception and find their symptoms worsen as they progress through their pregnancy. Pressure of the uterus on the rectum during the last trimester can also influence your bowel movements and worsen constipation.

Another contributing factor to constipation in pregnancy is from iron supplementation. If your health care provider recommended iron supplements, find a liquid form that is non-constipating. If you are anemic and low in iron during pregnancy you may also be low in vitamin-C, Vitamin-Bs and folate. Without sufficient vitamins like vitamin-C the body is unable to absorb iron. It is a great idea to eat vitamin-C rich foods like kiwi and oranges with iron rich foods like fresh spinach.

Regular Exercise

Movement and mild exercise assists in the elimination process. However, intense exercise can contribute to constipation if you are not eating water rich foods and drinking enough water.

Bacteria

Proper digestion and absorption of nutrients are affected by the amounts of probiotic bacteria or "friendly bacteria" in your intestinal tract. Not only do healthy colonies of probiotics assist in bowel functioning, but they also help prevent the more damaging and harmful pathogens from taking up residence. Patients who have had intestinal symptoms of gas, bloating, constipation, diarrhea, mucus, intestinal spasms, cramping and inflammation have had great improvement in intestinal health in only eight weeks after including probiotics in their diet. Sources of probiotics include sauerkraut, kefir, homemade yogurt and probiotic supplements. Kombucha tea is also a healthy probiotic source. However it has some caffeine, so it is not recommended while pregnant or nursing.

Quick Keys to Establishing Easy & Healthy Bowel Movements
- Create an early morning routine.
- Wake up around the same time each day.
- Brush the bacteria off your tongue and teeth.
- Drink a large glass of water after brushing.
- Let fruit be the first food you eat for the day.
- Eat your meals at regular times.
- Eat healthy, water rich foods. Eat fiber rich whole foods.
- Exercise regularly.

- Cultivate a positive mindset around bowel movements.
- Reduce stress.
- Stay hydrated throughout the day.
- Go to the bathroom whenever your body prompts you to go. Withholding a bowel movement creates stress in the digestive system and over time can cause compaction, pain and spasms.
- Create a consistent evening routine.
- Avoid eating three hours before you go to bed.
- Go to bed early and at the same time each night. A lack of sleep can cause stress hormones to be produced leading to colon disruptions
- Avoid long-term use of laxatives. Find natural solutions when possible.

Eat a Balanced Diet

Adequate nutrition during pregnancy is the single most important physical factor in determining the outcome of pregnancy.

~ Anne Frye

Scientists have documented that a lack of or an excess of certain nutrients during pregnancy has an effect on your baby's long-term health and genetics.

Prenatal nutrition is the foundation for the development of your baby in utero. It is very important during your pregnancy to eat a balanced diet for your health and the health of your baby. The best advice I can give you is to eat as much organic, whole, living, unprocessed foods as possible. The main point with your diet is to keep it balanced and to make sure that you have a wide range of foods that are full of healthy fats. Healthy eating is one of the most important gifts you can give to you and your baby.

154

Stress & Nutrition

Your baby eats what you eat. Which ever nutrients you are deficient in, your baby will be also be deficient in. If you are not obtaining the nutrients you need, some of the first symptoms you may experience include irritability, inability to respond to situations effectively, confusion, mood swings, anxiety, depression and frustration.

I know when I am feeling stressed, especially when I am busy with work, one of the first things I do is assess my recent water and nutritional intake. Here is a simple checklist I use in my mind:

- Have I had a glass of water in the last two hours?
- Have I eaten greens in a salad, green juice or a green smoothie in the last 24 hours?
- Have I eaten an avocado or consumed some coconut oil in the last 24 hours?
- Have I eaten at least three pieces of fruit in the last 24 hours?
- Have I consumed a healthy portion of protein in the last 24 hours?
- Have I eaten junk food within the last three hours?

I have noticed how essential green leafy foods are to my brain and mood. My husband is so familiar with this list that when I am feeling irritable or my brain isn't functioning optimally he offers to make me a green juice or a salad.

It is important to be aware of the significant relationship between stress and nutrition. In general, our adrenal glands produce a hormone called cortisol to assist the body to deal with stress and inflammation. Although cortisol is helpful in providing a necessary surge of energy in time of flight or fight, as well as brain stimulation for more intense awareness, cortisol reduces immune system activity to save energy for physical activity. Since cortisol is meant to be an emergency preparedness hormone, it is harmful to the body to have elevated or chronic production of it in our daily lives.

When there is inflammation in the body due to a consistently poor diet cortisol production becomes prolonged and contributes to a variety of symptoms and detrimental effects on the body. Some of these symptoms include tense nerves and muscles, ligament damage, mental and physical exhaustion, nerve pain, irritable bowel, leaky gut, hormonal imbalances, weight gain (especially around the abdomen), autoimmune disease, Candida, arthritis and hypoglycemia.

High levels of cortisol are also known to impede the body's ability to repair cellular damage, contribute to depression and emotional imbalances, suppress insulin production and affect your quality of sleep.

Stress & Junk Food Cravings

Excess cortisol also causes blood sugar levels to fluctuate triggering the body to crave foods high in fat, sugar and salt, which cause inflammation. Think about how many times you've turned to chocolate, ice cream or cookies when you've had a stressful day. Break the cycle of poor eating. Support yourself with healthy foods to undo the damage that both stress and poor eating habits cause in the body. A recent research study reported a higher risk of depression in association with consumption of fast foods such as hamburgers, sausages and pizza.[113]

Also be aware that cravings for certain foods occur not because of those foods but because of the nutrients within them. For example, craving chocolate can be due to a lack of magnesium and chromium in your diet.

Instead, consume greens, broccoli, nuts, legumes and fruit. For sugar and sweet cravings, try eating fish, eggs, dairy, nuts, whole grains, broccoli, spinach, cauliflower, cabbage, cranberries, raisins and yams. To satisfy a fatty food craving, ensure you are eating healthy fats such as avocado, hempseed nuts and coconut oil.

Foods that Contribute to Inflammation & Cellular Damage

White Sugar - White sugar can create havoc to your health. There are so many research studies on the detrimental effects of white sugar that it is a wonder why anyone would choose to consume it. Some significant effects of sugar in the body includes suppression of the immune system, hyperactivity, anxiety, loss of tissue elasticity, weakening eyesight, gastrointestinal disease, premature aging, obesity, autoimmune diseases, Candida growth, gallstones, hemorrhoids, varicose veins, tooth decay, toxemia during pregnancy, emphysema, damaging the pancreas, headaches and migraines, depression and a very long list of more health issues.[114] Excess sugar consumption can also affect fetal development.

Genetically Modified Foods - In recent animal studies, genetically modified (GM) foods have been linked to obesity, infertility, miscarriages, preterm labor, birth defects,[115] damage to the digestive system,[116] fetal exposure to pesticides,[117] mammary or liver tumors, disruption of the endocrine system and premature aging.[118] One of the best ways to avoid GM foods is to purchase locally grown organic foods. Remember, not all foods in your organic grocery store are organic. Do not rely on your grocer to label GM foods. Unless a non-organic product is labeled as non-GMO, it may very well be genetically modified if it contains the typical GM food items such as non-organic wheat, corn, soy, canola, sugar beets and corn derivatives. There is a new initiative by the Non-GMO Project to verify non-GMO foods. Visit www.nongmoproject.org for more information.

Soy & Soy Based Foods - Soy consumption has been linked to breast cancer, brain damage, infant abnormalities, thyroid disorders, kidney stones, immune system impairment, food allergies, infertility and hormone disruption.[119] Research studies suggest that the consumption of soybean related foods during pregnancy and while nursing exposes fetuses to phytoestrogens that affects the development of the fetus and the newborn.[120] It has also been suggested that drinking soymilk during pregnancy can cause a failure to produce breast milk. Since many infant formulas contain soy, if you choose not to breast feed, make sure to research formulas for your baby that are soy free.

Unnatural Oils - The problem with soybean oil, cottonseed oil, corn oil, canola oil, sunflower oil and other similar oils is that they have a high percentage of polyunsaturated fats (the most highly reactive type of fat), which leaves them prone to oxidation and free radical production when exposed to heat and light. The result of consuming these oils is damage to cells, depression to the immune system, inflammation and toxicity. Unfortunately, most processed foods contain these oils (salad dressing, mayo, margarine, breads, pastries, muffins, French fries, potato chips, canned meats, canned soups, cream substitutes, ice cream, roasted nuts, etc). Read labels or prepare your own meals to ensure your food does not contain these highly toxic oils.

Table Salt - Table salt is derived from chemically treated earth salt deposits that are devoid of additional minerals. In addition, anti-caking agents are added to salt to make ensure it flows freely without clumping. Iodine is also added to fortify salt. In contrast, high quality sea salt, like Celtic or Himalayan, is derived from evaporated seawater and can contain over 84 trace minerals. Since sea salt is not fortified with iodine, be sure to also consume kelp or dulse in your diet to obtain iodine if you consume sea salt. Salt and iodine are essential nutrients in your diet. However, excessive salt consumption is burdensome on the body.

White Flour - The detrimental effects of white flour on the body is well documented. Some of the symptoms that are commonly associated with consumption of white flour include depression, fatigue, intestinal bloating, diabetes, allergies, asthma, increased weight gain, hypoglycemia, brain fogginess, sleepiness, increased blood pressure, raised insulin levels, sluggish digestion, intestinal issues and more.

For the most part, the grain food supply also contains mycotoxins which are toxic chemical products produced by fungus. Mycotoxins are poisonous to the brain and nervous system and ultimately suppress immune function. Since there are very small amounts of nutrients remaining from the original grain in flour and it is highly toxic to the body, I recommend consuming whole grains.

Highly Processed Foods - Avoid commercial cereals, puff products like rice crackers, foods with a long shelf life (boxed foods, canned foods, TV dinners and highly processed meat products such as deli meat).

Microwaved Food - Microwaving food is a form of food irradiation that causes damage to the molecular structures of the food. Even more detrimental is heating food in plastic or with plastic film over top, as it releases carcinogenic toxins into your food. [121]

According to US researcher William Kopp, who reviewed results of Russian and German research, heating food in a microwave for human consumption:

- Created destabilization of active protein biomolecular compounds in prepared meats.
- Created cancer-causing agents in milk and cereal grains,
- Altered catabolic behavior of plant-alkaloids when raw, cooked or frozen vegetables were exposed for short periods,
- Created carcinogens in raw root vegetables,
- Vastly reduced the availability of essential minerals and vitamin complexes A, B, C and E. [122]

Absolutely never microwave breast milk or baby formula. Research studies have shown that microwaving breast milk destroys valuable antibodies, nutrients and disease-fighting agents in the breast milk. [123] In addition, "hot spots" from uneven heating can scald your baby.

I love the microwaved water experiment that a young girl submitted for her science fair project.[124] For her project she took filtered water and divided it into two parts. The first part she heated to boiling in a pan on the stove, and the second part she heated to boiling in a microwave. Then after cooling she used the cooled water to feed two identical plants to see if there would be any difference in the growth between the normal boiled water and the water boiled in a microwave. After nine days, the plant that received microwaved water was unhealthy and without foliage. Whereas the plant that received the non-microwaved water looked similar to the first day of the experiment with all of its leaves intact.

Summary of Foods to Avoid or Eliminate That Contribute to Cellular Damage

- Eliminate simple carbohydrates such as sugar, bread products and pasta made with white flour, pastries and white rice.
- Eliminate all GM foods such as non-organic wheat, corn, canola, sugarbeets and corn derivatives.
- Avoid processed foods from boxes or cans.
- Avoid microwaved food.
- Avoid deep fried foods such as French fries and potato chips.
- Avoid sugar-laden foods such as ice cream, cake, cookies and chocolate bars.
- Eliminate soy and soy based foods.
- Avoid store bought spreads, soups and sauces that contain preservatives and unhealthy oils.
- Avoid peanuts, as they are susceptible to a type of mold that produces mycotoxins called aflatoxins, which are carcinogenic and have been shown to affect human health and increase liver cancer mortality.

Foods that Support & Heal the Body

To neutralize free radical damage it is favorable to have an antioxidant system of vitamins, minerals, essential fatty acids and enzymes working for you. A diet that includes antioxidant rich, raw foods (such as avocado, sweet peppers, berries, melons, green leafy vegetables, oranges, tomatoes and pineapples) is key to radiating health from the inside out!

161

Fruit - A fabulous fuel that is great for reducing oxidative stress, fruit is packed with highly balanced water, minerals, vitamins and fiber. Fruit juices are not as healthy because of the lack of fiber, which slows down the absorption of sugar. However, you can create blended fruit smoothies or blended fruit juices, by simply blending the whole fruit rather than separating the juice from the fiber. It is also important to eat properly ripened fruit. Fruit that is not fully ripened takes more energy to digest because the body has to change it from starch to sugar.

Foods High in Folic Acid - The word folate is derived from foliage or leaves. The top foods high in folic acid include lentils and leafy greens such as fresh spinach and dark kale. Other great sources of greens high in folate are collards, romaine and dandelion. Fresh spinach and romaine are a great combination in salads. I like to put chopped kale into my soups at the end of cooking, so I don't damage the chlorophyll. Other cooked greens can be eaten as a simple side dish or added to soups. Broccoli is not only high in folic acid, but is a nutrient dense source of Vitamin C, beta-carotene, calcium and iron. Avocado is also an excellent source of folic acid. Greens are the star of the food world. Greens transform sunshine into vital nutrients such as proteins, vitamins, fats, hormones and micro-compounds micronutrients. Greens contain **all** essential vitamins, minerals and amino acids.

Whole Grains - Some of the best whole grains include quinoa, sprouted grain bread, bulgur wheat and brown rice. If you can eat gluten free I suggest that you give it a try. In the US, 1 in 133 people suffer from celiac disease and between 5% and 10% of all people may suffer from a gluten sensitivity of some form. Many people do not know they have sensitivity to gluten.

Gluten is a scientifically known hormone disruptor and it is also known to contribute to problems with conception. Gluten is found in barley, rye, oats and wheat. Sprouted or soaked grains have far less gluten than non-sprouted grains. Typically all wheat flour and products with wheat flour have not been sprouted. Gluten free foods include: wild rice, brown rice, quinoa, millet, amaranth and buckwheat.

Many people are not aware of this, but all grains and legumes in their dried form contain phytic acid, which is known to block absorption of minerals and proteins, leading to iron and calcium deficiencies, as well as other health issues. To prevent dietary deficiencies grains and legumes must be soaked, sprouted or fermented. These processes assist in the activation of the enzyme phytase, which neutralizes phytic acid to make them digestible and less stressful on the body.

Proteins - Make sure you consume a good balance of protein. Eggs are a good source of protein, vitamin B12, folate, lutein and choline. Organic and grain fed hens produce eggs that are higher in omega-3 fatty acids compared to non-organic eggs. Hemp seeds are an exceptional source of protein and they provide omega-3 and omega-6 fatty acids. They are also a good source of vitamin E, calcium, iron, phosphorus, magnesium, zinc, copper and manganese. Hemp seeds can be eaten alone or sprinkled on your yogurt, cereal or into sauces right before you serve.

Quinoa and chia seeds are complete proteins that have anti-inflammatory properties, support heart health, energize the body and stabilize blood sugar. Avocado is also a high quality, complete protein that offers the benefits of many vitamins, nutrients and essential fatty acids. Broccoli, spinach, romaine and kale are great protein-rich leafy vegetables. In addition, they supply your body with important vitamins, minerals and fiber.

Fish a good high protein food. Unfortunately, if it is wild fish, it most likely has high levels of mercury. However, Pacific Northwest fish tends to be much lower in mercury than other sources of fish. If the fish is farm-raised, high levels of antibiotics and dioxin may be present.

Iron - As pregnancy progresses, women need additional iron to support the growing fetus and placenta, and to support the brain development in the fetus. Iron deficiency anemia is one of the most common nutritional deficiencies during pregnancy. Eat iron-rich foods along with foods that contain vitamin C, which helps the body absorb the iron. Spinach, collard greens, kale, broccoli, peas, Brussels sprouts, bok choy and tomatoes contribute both iron and vitamin C to your diet. Ensure your prenatal vitamin includes a non-constipating iron supplement. In addition, you can also find a high quality liquid iron supplement to ensure your iron levels are met.

Large amounts of calcium hinder the absorption of iron; avoid high-calcium foods for a half hour before or after eating iron-rich foods. Be aware that gluten intolerance and Celiac disease can also prevent the absorption of iron and can contribute to iron deficiency. Parasites are another source of iron deficiency. If you suspect parasites, get tested.

Per 100g serving, some of the best vegetarian sources of iron are:
- Hemp seeds provide 128% of your daily requirement (4/5 cup)
- Raw pumpkin seeds provide 83% of your daily requirement (¾ cup)
- Parsley gives you 35% of your daily requirement (1¾ cup)
- Raw hazelnuts yield 26% of your daily requirement (¾ cup)
- Molasses 25% of your daily requirement (just under 1/3 cup)
- Raw almonds allow for 21% of your daily requirement (just under ¾ cup)
- Cooked lentils offer 19% of your daily requirement (½ cup)

- Cooked chickpeas gives you 16% of your daily requirement (2/3 cup)
- Chopped raw kale yields 9% of your daily requirement (just under ¾ cup)
- Cooked quinoa provides 8% of your daily requirement (just over ½ cup)

Per 100g serving, some of the best meat sources of iron are:
- Braised chuck beef offers 21% of your daily requirement
- Roasted boneless leg of lamb provides 10% of your daily requirement
- Most cooked fish provides 9% of your daily requirement
- Scrambled eggs offers 7% of your daily requirement (just under ½ cup)
- Cheddar cheese 5% of your daily requirement (¾ cup)[125]

Fat - Essential Fatty Acids (EFAs) are necessary fats in our diet. EFA imbalances and deficiencies place immense stress on the body and brain. Ultimately, the body requires EFAs to support a multitude of functions including, cardiovascular, immune, reproductive, digestive and nervous systems.

During gestation, omega-3 fatty acid consumption is important to prevent prenatal depression[126] and to assist in a healthy pregnancy. Fetuses and breast-fed infants also require an adequate supply of EFAs through the mother's dietary intake, as they are critical for brain development. [127]

EFA supplementation may help prevent or treat ADD, ADHD,[128] depression, decreased memory and mental abilities, mental disorders, cognitive decline, skin disorders, poor vision, diabetes, arthritis, diminished immune function, increased triglycerides and 'bad' cholesterol (LDL) levels, impaired membrane function, hypertension, irregular heart beat, colorectal cancer, breast cancer, prostate cancer, learning disorders, menstrual pain and menopausal discomfort.[129] [130]

There are two essential fatty acids:

- Alpha-Linolenic acid (LNA) or omega-3 is found in abundance in hemp seeds, flax seeds, pumpkin seeds, walnuts, avocado, fish oil, krill oil, algae and dark green leaves.
- Linoleic acid (LA) or omega-6 is found in abundance in avocado, hemp seeds, walnuts, pumpkin seeds, sesame seeds, sunflower seeds and flax seeds.

Since humans cannot synthesize EFAs they must be obtained through diet in the proper ratio of omega-6 to omega-3 fatty acids somewhere between 1:1 and 4:1. To maintain a balance between omega-6 and 3s, reduce consumption of processed foods and polyunsaturated vegetable oils such as corn, cottonseed, sunflower and soy.

Avocado is a nutrition rich superfood that is high in fiber, potassium, folate, essential fatty acids and vitamins A, B6, C, D, E and K. Among fruits, avocado is exceptional for the quantity and quality of its protein and unlike most plant sources it is a complete protein. Eating more avocado is a great way to access antioxidants to help prevent diseases such as arthritis, cancer and heart disease.

Other healthy sources of healthy fat include almonds, sunflower seeds, almond butter, hazelnuts, coconut oil, low mercury fish (shrimp, prawn, rainbow trout, sole, Atlantic mackerel and pacific north west albacore tuna and salmon), krill oil and cold pressed oils. Do not cook cold pressed oils. Instead use them in dressings or in a cold sauce.

High heat denatures and destroys linolenic acid, so make sure you consume unheated or uncooked sources of essential fatty acids. If you are going to cook with oil, coconut oil is the most stable at high temperatures. However, coconut oil does not contain omega-3 fatty acids. It is, however, one of the best sources of medium chain fatty acids, so make sure you consume some uncooked coconut oil, too. I often finish my soups with coconut oil by adding a couple of tablespoons once my soup is done cooking.

Organic vs. Non-organic

There is a lot of debate surrounding organic vs. non-organic food. Both sides have interesting arguments, but the organic side wins out with me. My first choice in food is to grow it myself or buy from local organic farmers. My second choice is my local organic grocer. However, I'd rather eat healthy, alive, non-organic food instead of old, wilted, sickly or rotting organic food.

I also don't buy everything organic. Sometimes organic is not available or items may be too expensive. For example, at times I may purchase non-organic avocados and oranges. However, I feel it's important to buy organic greens, root veggies, corn, apples, pears and meat. My suggestion is to do your own research, follow your instincts and work within your budget.

Write a Weekly Menu & Grocery List

As a child my family's menu consisted of two choices: take it or leave it.

~ Buddy Hackett

Weekly menu planning is a great way to save time and money in the kitchen. If you haven't tried organizing your week this way, give it a try. Having a menu plan organized for the week frees you up from having to figure it out as you go along. When it is integrated with your grocery list, you'll be sure to

167

have what you need without having to take another trip to the store. In addition, when you buy only what you need for the week, you are more likely to not have any rotting wasted produce left over. Every perishable item that goes unused is money in the garbage.

Planning meals in advance is also a great way to plan to eat healthier. Type up a list of ingredients you'd normally purchase and print off copies to be used when making your list, that way you just have to check off the items you actually need or cross out the stuff you don't need. Your list will change over time and you will become more efficient as the weeks go by. If you don't like to plan seven days in advance, try menu planning for four days.

Have a list of favorite recipes on your fridge as a reminder of the meals you might like to make when you are doing your menu planning. You can add to the list as you find great recipes. If a menu plan works successfully for you, keep it and reuse it, saving you even more time. You may even come up with four weekly plans that you can rotate for a few months.

Remember to also plan seasonally. In the winter months, you are not going to eat all the same meals you made in the summer. For those who've implemented menu planning for a year, reusing the previous years plans will be a breeze. The key to menu planning is to keep it diverse and filled with healthy food you know you are going to love!

Sunday Prep Days

Sundays are a great day to prep food you may be using in the coming week. Make your salads for the next few days. It's a great way to ensure you eat them. Wash, chop and store all your ingredients in separate containers on Sunday and Wednesday; you'd be surprised how fast making dinner will be.

Become a Gourmet Chef for a Meal

One cannot think well, love well, sleep well, if one has not dined well.

~ Virginia Woolf

Although cooking may be the last thing you want to do while you are pregnant, it can be a wonderful way to help alleviate stress and to bond with your partner. Choose a meal that is new and interesting before you head into the kitchen and make sure that you will enjoy making it.

When you look at becoming a gourmet chef for a meal, you consider the many different benefits that are attributed to cooking:

- *A healthier choice* - Obviously, cooking is much healthier for you than eating take out and you can really enjoy the benefits of choosing fresh produce and the right serving sizes.

- *Gives you a boost of confidence* - Choosing to be a gourmet chef for a meal can give you a huge boost of confidence in your abilities.

- *Reduces stress* - Cooking can reduce stress if you allow your mind to be present with the tasks at hand. Enjoy the creativity in the moment as you prepare and cook food!

- *Provides time to bond* - Either you or your partner can take the role of chef or sous-chef. Cooking together can be an opportunity to talk, laugh and just enjoy each other's company.

- *Saves money* - Finally, if you find you spend a lot of money eating out, cooking at home will help you cut your spending.

169

Find Natural Solutions to Medical Issues

Each year approximately 2.2 million US hospital patients experience
adverse drug reactions to prescribed medications.

~ Dr. Gary Null (et al), Death by Medicine

There is a growing concern among health practitioners of the increasing number of women who are taking pharmaceuticals during their pregnancy. In a large US study, researchers estimated that 64% of expecting women have been prescribed one or more drugs during their pregnancy.[131]

Due to the harmful and stressful effects of prescribed drugs on fetal development and maternal health, researchers have recently begun conducting studies on non-pharmacological interventions for the effective reduction of stress, anxiety and depression. Studies revealed that mind-body therapies not only showed reduction of stress, anxiety, and depression,[132] but also revealed benefits of better sleep, shorter length of birthing, less instrument-assisted births and higher birth weight.[133] Beneficial and effective non-drug, mind-body therapies during pregnancy include:

- Mindful and gentle prenatal yoga
- Prenatal education classes
- Mindfulness practice such as meditation
- Visualization
- Hypnotherapy, Hypnobirthing and Hypnobabies
- Emotional Freedom Technique (EFT)
- Tai Chi
- Acupuncture and acupressure

Fetal Health

We know that the chemical influence of cigarettes, alcohol and recreational drugs alter the DNA of fetuses. Why is it such a stretch for the medical community and the public to make the leap that prescription drugs chemically alter the DNA of fetuses? Drugs that may be of some benefit to the mother can deform, kill or alter the DNA of fetuses causing irreversible damage and a lifetime of mental or physical trauma. It is key to educate your self about the risks of pharmaceuticals to your baby.

Research often looks at the major effects of chemical drugs on a fetus and overlooks or fails to study the less perceptible long-term effects on fetuses. I remember recently reading in a chat room various women who were sharing that their baby's were born normal even though they took antidepressants. What these women do not yet know is what kind of effect their antidepressants have had on the long-term health of their babies. In addition, there are also many online stories of women sharing about the birth defects they believed resulted from SSRI antidepressants.

Ultimately, there have been no adequate and well-controlled studies to determine the delayed, long-term effects of any medication on pregnant women, or on the neurological or physical development of the children exposed to pharmaceuticals in utero. Health and developmental issues such as autism and ADHD are usually not detected before 24 months. Some symptoms of prenatal damage, such as diabetes, obesity and heart disease do not surface until the teens or even adulthood.

Scientists are just beginning to look at the long-term side effects of pharmaceuticals, even common ones. Research is beginning to reveal that pharmaceuticals can alter DNA, not only while you are taking them, but also

171

long after you've stopped taking them.[134] These persistent genetic changes are not only passed on from you and your partner to your child when you conceive but can also alter your baby's DNA if you are taking them while pregnant. You may recall that any prescriptions you've had filled in the last decade have warning labels to not take them if pregnant unless under the supervision of a physician.

The FDA has only approved a dozen pharmaceuticals to be used during pregnancy and all are related to gestation, birthing or nausea. Of these approved drugs, the FDA has not determined if that drug is free from harming or injuring the woman taking it or her baby. Almost all medication is being used in the dark, without adequate testing. I was shocked to learn that "...the FDA has no way of knowing the true incidence of risk to the patient because there is no law or regulation that requires a doctor or other health care provider to report the adverse drug reaction to the FDA, even if the patient dies." [135]

In 2004, a study determined that 37.8% of women who were prescribed drugs during pregnancy, were given pharmaceuticals that have known side effects to the fetus in animal studies and there have been no human studies.[136] If you are prescribed medication, make sure you discuss all possible side effects with your doctor. Also, do a search online for side effects before you begin any medication.

Antidepressants

Various studies suggest that fetal exposure to SSRI antidepressants may include side effects such as spontaneous abortions and miscarriage,[137] low birth weight, fetal death, infant death,[138] prolonged hospitalization[139] and fetal birth defects[140] with long-term health implications for infants and young children. One study found that expecting women who took anti-depressants during their last trimester were over five times more likely to birth babies born with persistent pulmonary hypertension,[141] which causes damage to the lungs, high blood pressure, and restricted oxygen levels in the blood. The lack of oxygen in the blood leads to stress on the brain, kidneys and liver.

Researchers in other studies found that SSRIs increased the risk of a baby developing autism spectrum disorder,[142] clubfoot, heart defects,[143] oral cleft, craniosynostosis[144] and developmental delays.

"There is no evidence that SSRIs in pregnancy improve maternal or infant health, and substantive evidence that they pose a risk to the fetus. Thus the harms exceed the benefits in this setting."[145] There are even studies that suggest that SSRI antidepressants failed to differ in comparison to placebos with people who are moderately depressed. Even with those who are severely depressed, the effectiveness of antidepressants is relatively small in comparison with placebos.[146] No studies have been done yet on father's use of SSRIs prior to conception.

Natural Solutions

There are risks to your baby if you are stressed and depressed while pregnant. However, there are greater risks to taking antidepressants and other pharmaceuticals as well. The key is to work with a health professional to heal what is at the root of your stress and depression rather than taking a pill that may only mask the underlying issue. Whenever possible utilize the suggested mind-body practices, nutritional strategies and relaxation techniques offered throughout this book to reduce your stress, anxiety and depression naturally.

EFT is at the top of my list because of its incredible results. Ensure you are meeting your basic prenatal needs for nutrition, sleep, rest, exercise and emotional support.

Life Saving Drugs

Although there may be side effects to pharmaceuticals, under certain circumstances prescribed medication and medical intervention may be necessary to assist in saving the life of a woman or fetus in emergency situations or chronic disease. Please consult your health care professional for any medical advice.

Avoid Stimulants

Caffeine is an example of a toxic stimulant. The burst of energy, or "lift" we feel after drinking coffee, is the result of the body being stimulated to rid itself of the caffeine. Likewise, sugar is a stimulant and a toxin because it contains no nutrition and must be combined with other nutrients, such as calcium from the body's stores, to eliminate it from the body. Toxins and most stimulants are negatives to the body. The energy required to eliminate them comes from the body's energy and mineral stores, and not from the stimulating substances.

~ Ron Garner, Conscious Health

During pregnancy many women experience fatigue, brain fog and a lack of energy because of the nutritional and energetic resources required to grow a new being. When faced with a sleepy brain most of the general population tends to use stimulants to wake them up and get them going. Unfortunately,

174

stimulants don't fix the root problem, instead they contribute to overall stress and fatigue by taxing the nervous and adrenal systems. In reality, stimulants can amplify the symptoms of stress that we experience, hinder our ability to relax and prevent us from sleeping soundly.

Since stimulants are harmful to a growing fetus, expecting women need to address the issue at the root. When you need extra sleep, find the time to have a nap or go to bed earlier. Some weeks of my pregnancy required 10 to 12 hours of sleep each night, while at other times, 8 hours was sufficient. To address the root issue of brain fog, ensure you consume essential fatty acids and good fats such as avocado, coconut oil and hemp seed nuts. Also, avoid overeating and heavy carbohydrate meals, such as pasta, that are difficult to digest.

Caffeine is a major stimulant that you should avoid during pregnancy. Not only does it keep you feeling jittery throughout the day, it also raises your heart rate and your blood pressure, which can be very detrimental to both you and your child. Too much caffeine consumption can block your body from absorbing and properly using calcium and iron. In addition, caffeine is a diuretic, which means that you will lose fluids in your body faster and can become dehydrated.

Studies have indicated that caffeine can increase your baby's heart rate,[147] can affect heart development and function,[148] may prevent important nutrients from getting to your baby,[149] may inhibit fetal skeletal growth[150] and affects your baby's neuroendocrine system[151] (which controls reactions to stress and regulates digestion, the immune system, mood and emotions and hormones).

Most women are aware of the caffeine in coffee and black or green tea, but there are also large amounts of caffeine in energy drinks and most brands of pop. Avoid pop and energy drinks as the ingredients tend to include caffeine, sugar, dangerous artificial sweeteners and harmful chemical stabilizers. Reported side effects of consuming energy drinks have included anxiety, hypertension, sleep disruption, strokes, seizures, heart palpitations and even sudden death.[152]

With women who drink up to two cups or more a day of caffeinated beverages, the likelihood of miscarrying can increase greatly and this puts both you and your child at risk.[153] In addition, caffeine is also a stimulant known to deplete the adrenals and result in long-term energy loss. Avoid it completely. Instead, choose decaffeinated drinks or stick to the best liquid you can provide for your baby: fresh, clean water.

In addition to caffeine, which is a common stimulant, there are several other types of herbal stimulants that you should avoid during pregnancy:

- Arbor Vitae, which is a stimulant used for menstruation.
- Barberry, which will stimulate uterine contractions.
- Beth Root, can be used but only during childbirth as it stimulates the uterus.
- Black and Blue Cohosh, can lead to miscarriage and preterm childbirth.
- Bloodroot, another uterine stimulant, bloodroot can cause vomiting.
- Broom, avoid this herb to prevent uterine contractions.
- Cotton Root, can cause preterm childbirth.
- Devil's Claw, is a source of oxytocin, which causes birthing to start.
- Lady's Mantle, it can be used in childbirth to increase uterine activity.
- Liferoot, not only is it a stimulant but it also crosses the placenta and can be toxic to your fetus.
- Mugwart, another stimulant that can cause birth defects in your

infant.

- Pennyroyal, both the American and European varieties can lead to childbirth and should be avoided. In addition, the stimulant can cause birth defects.

- Peruvian Bark, this is used to treat malaria but it can be very toxic to the infant and can lead to blindness.

- Rue, can cause preterm childbirth and miscarriage.

- Tansy, another stimulant that can cause birth defects in your infant.

- Wild Yam, another uterine stimulant, wild yam can be used during childbirth but not at any other time.

Notes: Before you use any type of herb or drug, check with your health care practitioner to make sure that there are no negative side effects for you or your baby.

Eliminate Recreational Drugs

You own yourself, so if you want to do something that destroys yourself, go ahead. Just don't harm others when you do.

~ *Jim Goebel*

Your baby experiences every chemical you ingest or inhale. The difference between you and your baby is that you are fully developed; your baby is growing from a dot to a seven-pound baby. Fetal development is a constant chemical process that leaves the fetus susceptible to chemical influences. Any chemical interference adversely affects your baby's physical and mental development.

Various research studies suggest that the effects of marijuana use on fetal development during pregnancy significantly relates to post-birth issues such as difficulty sleeping,[154] impulsivity, hyperactivity, child behavioral issues[155] and depressive symptoms[156] later in development. Essentially, for your baby's brain and developing nervous system, it is safer for you to not use marijuana while you are pregnant and breastfeeding.

Using other recreational drugs or solvents to get high has devastating and detrimental effects on a baby's development and can lead to premature birth, severe birth defects, sensitivity to sound and light, mental retardation and even death.

If you need assistance and support to stop using drugs while pregnant, contact a physician who can recommend treatment, support and programs.

Eliminate Alcohol

Pleasure which must be enjoyed at the expense of another's pain,
can never be enjoyed by a worthy mind.

~ *Augustine J. Duganne*

Developing babies are incredibly vulnerable to the effects of alcohol. At one time, most people, including doctors, used to think that drinking while pregnant was not a problem. In the last few decades increasing research has revealed that any amount of alcohol compromises the development of a fetus, especially in the first trimester.

If you'd like to see some sobering images, do an online search for "fetal alcohol syndrome brain" and click on images to view the devastating effects of alcohol on the fetal brain. Many drinking people say they don't have a drinking problem. A women's attachment to the need to drink or the justification of drinking while pregnant may reveal just how addicting a substance like alcohol can be. Some of the potential side effects[157] of drinking alcohol while pregnant include:

- Physical deformities
- Behavioral problems
- Mental development issues
- Fetal Alcohol Spectrum Disorder
- Smaller birth weight
- Smaller brain and head development
- Unusually thin upper lip
- Brain damage
- Hearing and vision problems
- Sensitivity to light, touch or sound
- Kidney and bladder problems
- Depression
- Attention and learning difficulties
- And much more

If you self medicate with alcohol to reduce stress, there are many alternatives in this book to assist you to reduce stress. If you are having difficulty quitting drinking while pregnant, obtain medical assistance in combination with a support group or counseling. Give your baby the gift of being alcohol free. I also highly recommend Allen Carr's *Easyway to Stop Drinking*.

Quit Smoking While Pregnant

I'm more proud of quitting smoking than of anything else
I've done in my life, including winning an Oscar.

~ Christine Lahti

Smoking cigarettes are a major stress on the body. Ironically, smoking is one of the ways that smokers deal with stress. The main reason that smokers feel stress relief is because the nicotine causes the brain to release chemicals that make them feel better. However, the feeling is temporary and smoking only compounds physical stress on the body. Since smoking does not solve problems, it is important to resolve the underlying cause of the stress. Studies have shown that giving up smoking lowers stress levels after quitting.

Why is Smoking Harmful?

Cigarette smoke contains highly toxic and deadly poisons. There are over 4,000 chemicals in cigarette smoke. These chemicals include carbon monoxide, cyanide, arsenic, strychnine, formaldehyde, methanol, acetylene, ammonia and acetone. Many of these chemicals are known to cause cancer and do other harmful damage to the lungs and organs.

Diseases and disorders caused by smoking include abdominal aortic aneurysm, acute myeloid leukemia, cataract, COPD, coronary heart disease, infertility, peptic ulcer disease, periodontitis, pneumonia, stroke and cancers of the bladder, cervix, esophagus, kidney, larynx, lung, mouth, pancreas, stomach and throat.[158]

Nicotine itself is a dangerous and poisonous chemical. Not only is it addicting, it also affects blood pressure and pulse rate putting stress on the heart.

Why is Smoking Harmful for Babies?

Not only are cigarette smoke and nicotine stressful on your body, they are also highly stressful and harmful to a developing fetus. There have been cases where young children suffer from nicotine poisoning after chewing on nicotine patches or gum.

Studies have found that cigarette smoking and second hand smoke are known to have an effect on babies before they are born. The chemicals you inhale enter your blood stream and pass on to the baby through the placenta.[159] When you smoke or are exposed to second-hand smoke while pregnant:

- You put your pregnancy at risk for vaginal bleeding, placental abruption, placenta previa, premature birth, miscarriage, birth complications and stillbirth.[160]

- Your baby gets less oxygen and nutrients, which may cause slowed growth and less weight gain for the baby. Babies born with a lower-than-average birth weight tend to have more health problems.

- You expose your baby to over 4,000 chemicals found in tobacco smoke, which interfere with the many natural chemical processes needed to grow a fertilized egg into a trillion celled little baby.

- Your baby's health may be compromised for life with immunity issues, learning disabilities and breathing problems.[161 162 163]

Quitting Smoking

Quitting smoking may be challenging for a short amount of time, but it is definitely worth it for the long-term health of you and your baby.

Once you stop smoking, nicotine withdrawal lasts a couple of weeks. Knowing that you will experience symptoms helps to prepare to live through them. Some of the common and temporary withdrawal symptoms that you may experience when you quit smoking include constipation, lightheadedness, headaches, sleep problems, nausea, decreased heart rate, depression, craving for cigarettes, irritability, increased appetite, anxiety and difficulty thinking.

Wearing patches or chewing nicotine gum may not be the healthiest solution, as the presence of nicotine poses a potential risk to the fetus's long-term health. However, researchers suggest that nicotine replacements are far better than smoking due to the hundreds of harmful chemicals in cigarettes.

When you quit smoking try to avoid habit triggering situations and behaviors you associate with smoking. Habit urges can last up to a year, so it is important to create new habits, activities and lifestyle choices that foster non-smoking as part of your long-term plan. Some positive activities include learning a new skill, exploring a hobby, doing fun activities, taking a yoga class, going for a walk or reading a book.

Creating a Smoke-Free Environment

Second hand smoke also places a prenatal baby at risk for preterm birth, reduced birth weight, respiratory distress and newborn complications.[164] Avoid second-hand smoke by choosing smoke free restaurants and by making your home and car smoke-free spaces. Be firm with your family and friends about not smoking around you. Explain to them how important it is that you and your baby have smoke-free air.

Recommendations

If you need help quitting smoking I highly recommend reading Allen Carr's *Easyway to Stop Smoking: Be a Happy Non-smoker for the Rest of Your Life*. Many people have also had success with EFT, hypnosis and acupuncture.

Avoid Exposure to EMF's & Microwave Frequencies

Cells in the body react to EMFs as potentially harmful, just like to other environmental toxins, including heavy metals and toxic chemicals. The DNA in living cells recognizes electromagnetic fields at very low levels of exposure; and produces a biochemical stress response. The scientific evidence tells us that our safety standards are inadequate, and that we must protect ourselves from exposure to EMF due to power lines, cell phones and the like, or risk the known consequences. The science is very strong and we should sit up and pay attention.

~ Martin Blank, PhD

What is an Electromagnetic Field?

"Electromagnetic field" (EMF) is a term that increasing numbers of people are becoming familiar with due to the large number of cell phones, computers and Wi-Fi that permeate our daily lives. The term itself refers to a type of radiation that is caused by a magnetic, electric, high frequency or radio wave. It is also known as electro-smog and it is a problem that affects everyone. Studies have reported that every house in North America has 81% wireless penetration, which is a major contributor of EMF radiation.

Although EMFs affect everyone differently, and research is still being done on the effects of the radiation, there have been studies that link EMF radiation to infertility,[165] childhood leukemia, cancer, headaches, allergic and inflammatory responses, miscarriages,[166] chronic depression, insomnia and heart arrhythmias. Scientists are aware of the additional sensitivity of children, pregnant women and people with immune deficiencies to both EMFs and radio frequencies. They suggest that the standards set in North America do not provide adequate protection and need to be reevaluated.

In today's world, it can be very difficult to prevent EMFs, but there are ways that you can avoid being overexposed to them:

1. *Avoid sources of dirty electricity* such as microwave ovens, electric toothbrushes, fluorescent lighting, dimmer switches, hydro sub-stations and many other items that are electrical. Never use a plasma screen television as they emit a very high level of radiation. Instead use an LCD television. When you are not using an appliance, unplug it since this will cut down on the amount of EMF smog in your home. Avoid using cordless phones or cell phones for long periods and cut down on unnecessary computer time. If you use a baby monitor once your baby is born, keep it on the opposite side of the room from your baby.

2. *Avoid wireless Internet cafes.* Also avoid Wi-Fi hotspots in public areas and schools, especially if you find you are more sensitive.

3. *Be mindful where you sleep.* Avoid sleeping in rooms that share a wall with a smart meter, gas meter or that contain wireless electronics. Make sure devices such as electronic alarm clocks and power adapters are at least five feet from your body. If you can, make

your bedroom an appliance free room since these electric machines generate an EMF, even while off, and can affect your sleep patterns.

4. *Avoid living near cell towers and high-tension power lines* as they have been linked to major health conditions.

5. *Avoid using your cell phone in vehicles* such as buses, cars and elevators, as the metal of the vehicle magnifies and accelerates the radiation from your phone's antenna by up to ten times.

To help your body cope with EMF stress, eat a healthy balanced diet, connect with the earth more, spend time in nature, laugh, have fun, eliminate unnecessary stress and avoid unnecessary exposure to electronics and wireless devices. Go barefoot on the earth when you can to help release and ground any EMF charge that has built up in your body. If you can't go barefoot, wear shoes with leather soles.

Avoid Exposure to Geopathic Stress

Stressful effects upon human health, caused by abnormal fields associated with a particular geographical region, are referred to as "geopathic stress." Studies in Germany and England have produced evidence which suggests that geopathic stress may not only contribute to the production of illness, but that such stresses may hinder the effective treatment of diseases as well.

~ Richard Gerber, M.D.

Due to the rotation of the metal core in the center of the earth, the planet naturally generates and radiates electromagnetic networks of energy. However, distortions and irregularities in the earth's magnetic field can occur when they come into contact with subterranean water, mineral concentrations and fault lines. All living organisms, including humans, are affected by these distortions when they are located in the same area where the organism resides or sleeps. The earth energy networks all differ: some beneficial, some neutral and some extremely harmful. The harmful earth energies cause stress and damage to health and some can even contribute to life threatening diseases.

Not all organisms are affected the same way. For example, the energies that are harmful to humans are also harmful to dogs, horses, fish and trees. However, these same energies are beneficial to other organisms such as ants and cats.

The negative effects of these distortions are known as geopathic stress. The word 'geopathic' comes from two Greek words: the word "geo" that translates to "of the earth" and the word "pathos" translates into "disease." Although well known in Europe, North Americans are relatively in the dark about the effects of geopathic stress on their health. Unfortunately, like all energy, geopathic energy zones are invisible to the eye, but its effects can be seen in nature and in human health.

To find people who are properly trained to detect and correct these energy zones do an online search for keywords such as "geopathic stress" and "dowsing." If you have access to people who are skilled at detecting geopathic zones, the technology to prevent harmful earth energies or geopathic stress is fairly simple and often involves the installation of crystals, copper or brass around the home.

Geopathic stress can result in health complications, sensitivities, body specific injuries and diseases, migraines, difficulty sleeping and much more. A book by Käthe Bachler entitled *Earth Radiation*, demonstrates clearly that we should take geobiological influences on health very seriously. She has dowsed over 3,000 apartments in 14 countries and interviewed 11,000 people. She concluded that 95% of the 'problem' children she investigated slept in beds or worked at desks that were placed at zones exposed to harmful geopathic energies. She also checked a sample of 500 cancer cases; everyone was found to be sleeping over harmful earth radiation.

Avoid Sitting for Long Periods of Time

Even if people meet the current recommendation of 30 minutes of physical activity on most days each week, there may be significant adverse metabolic and health effects from prolonged sitting -- the activity that dominates most people's remaining "non-exercise" waking hours.

~ Neville Owen, The University of Queensland[167]

Sitting for long periods of time causes stress on the body and can play havoc with people's health. Research studies indicate that sitting shuts down the circulation of lipase, which is a fat absorbing enzyme. This lack of circulation can lead to obesity, heart disease and other health conditions. Scientists have discovered that the antidote to this isn't exercise. The solution is the simple act of standing, as it encourages the circulation of lipase, which triggers the body to process fat and cholesterol.[168] The more total time you spend standing is more important than the amount of exercise you do. So make sure you take standing breaks frequently throughout the day.

Sitting too long can also contribute to problems in your wrist, muscles, spine, hips and shoulders especially if you are sitting in front of a computer using a mouse. Although I mentioned that exercise wasn't helpful in the circulation of lipase, it is important for overall health of muscles, joints and connective tissue. Exercise also improves mood, boosts energy, delivers oxygen and nutrients to the tissues, helps the cardiovascular system work more efficiently, promotes sleep and provides much more benefit to physical, mental and emotional health.

Eyestrain is also associated with sitting to long in front of computers and can contribute to headaches, blurred vision and other visual symptoms. Taking breaks gives your eyes a micro-vacation from the arm's length field of vision we get locked into while focusing on a screen. A very simple exercise to give the eyes a break is to scan the room on objects at varying distances and with varying textures. Keep your eyes moving and only glance at objects for a few seconds. Do this for at least two minutes.

Another factor of sitting too long is the formation or the worsening of vein issues such as varicose or spider veins. Varicose veins occur when healthy vein walls become weak and the vein enlarges. Although the exact cause of varicose veins has not been established, there are certain risk factors that are associated. Some of the risk factors for varicose veins include hormonal changes, wearing tight fitting clothing, injury to the veins, exposure to ultra-violet rays, liver disease, a lack of circulation, constipation and more.

To prevent varicose and spider veins:

- Avoid crossing your legs and ankles while seated.

- Ensure your sitting posture has your legs at a 90-degree angle.

- Take frequent breaks from sitting and get up and move around for at least five minutes.

- Avoid wearing tight-fitting clothing that constricts the waist, groin or legs while seated.

- Eat a healthy diet rich in living foods that are high in fiber, vitamin E, vitamin C and selenium. Vitamin E offers many benefits to your health, including improving circulation and helps prevent and correct damage to veins. Selenium assists to keep the walls of veins elastic. Avocados are highly recommended for varicose veins because they are so rich in vitamin E, C and B6, as well as fiber, potassium and copper.

- Exercise to help prevent damage. If you don't have a regular exercise plan, implement a walk everyday for at least 20 minutes to ensure you circulate your blood. Other safe exercises for pregnant women include prenatal yoga, swimming and low impact dance.

Avoid Major Renovations

I'm picturing what it's like every time you renovate.
There's a big hole in the wall and two paramedics.

~ Jill says to Tim, from TV's Home Improvement

We have all seen the magic transformations on home renovation shows. The reality is far less glamorous as major renovations can be stressful at the best of times. During pregnancy, renovations can be a source of unnecessary stress for mom, dad and baby. Make sure you are aware of potential renovation challenges like additional expenses or delays that may arise. Also, ensure that renovations don't create tension and distract either of you from prenatal preparations and connecting with each other.

Limit your exposure to renovation noise, as the sounds in a women's environment are directly experienced by the developing fetus and have been shown to affect heart rate. Research has also revealed that excessive noise in living and working conditions can cause premature birth, birth defects and low birth weight in babies.[169] [170]

Another study discovered that mothers who were exposed to occupational noise in the range of 85 to 95 dB during pregnancy gave birth to babies with a three-fold increase in the risk of having high-frequency hearing loss.[171] Bursts of noise have also been shown to increase stress levels in fetuses of animals. Offspring whose mothers had been stressed with noise were more distractible and had lower motor maturity than offspring of undisturbed gestations.[172] Another study showed higher rates of abnormal and disturbed behavior with offspring who were prenatally stressed.[173]

If renovating, minimize your exposure to chemicals and organic solvents during pregnancy. Toxins such as Volatile Organic Compounds (VOCs) can off-gas from paint, flooring, particleboard, stains, varnishes, plywood, carpeting, insulation and other building products. Since off-gassing continues for years, they can affect your health long after construction has been completed.

VOCs are stored in body fat, so once they are in your system, they can lead to serious health problems over time. Increased risks of major fetal malformations are associated with prenatal exposure to organic solvents.[174] Buy paint, stains and sealers that have low to no VOCs. Do not store containers of paints and solvents inside your home. Instead store them in a shed or garage that is not attached to the house.

In addition, if you have walls with lead paint, sanding them to paint over them can create small particles that end up in carpets, furniture or cracks in the hardwood. Lead is extremely harmful to your baby. If you are going to repaint, do a lead strip test to make sure there isn't any lead in the old paint on the wall.

If renovations are necessary, see if you can move into a small apartment or stay with a relative or a friend until they are completed. Make sure you leave some time for off-gassing of volatiles.

Refrain From Watching Scary Films

It's not scary to make a horror film because you
get to pull back the curtain and see that none of it's real.
When you're watching one, the terror bombards you.

~ Josh Hartnett

Watching scary thrillers or horror films affects your brain in negative ways such as creating images to feed anxious thoughts and fears, raising blood pressure and contributing to nightmares and sleep issues.

Using MRI neuroimaging technology, researchers have demonstrated that during scary video scenes,[175] or while exposed to disturbing images,[176] the amygdala in the brain becomes activated with fear. This sets off a cascade of chemical processes that result in a stress response that spikes adrenaline and cortisol levels. We know that stress and cortisol secretion has adverse effects on a women's body and the fetus.

Although your conscious mind knows you are watching a horror film, your subconscious mind doesn't differentiate between what is real and what is imaginary. The subconscious reacts automatically to artificial stimuli with stress hormones as though it is your own experience.

When conditions are presented that are similar to the storyline of a horror movie you've watched, such as being at home alone during a storm or hearing a loud noise, your subconscious becomes activated and triggers an automatic fear-stress response and you may not even know why.

For example, many people who have watched the movie Jaws, have found themselves terrified to swim in open bodies of water for fear of sharks. The learned conditioned fear response is a function of perceived survival.[177]

Avoid Watching Birthing Shows That Depict Traumatic Births

I swear it traumatised me to this day. I haven't had children and now I can't look at anything to do with childbirth. It absolutely disgusts me.

~ Helen Mirren, (on watching an educational birthing film as a schoolgirl)

If you skipped over the section on refraining from watching scary films, review it because the same conditioning that occurs while watching horror films, also occurs while watching traumatic events during pregnancy and birthing. The last thing you need is to consciously or subconsciously link birth with trauma or emergency procedures.

Watching negative and traumatic shows about childbirth seeds your subconscious with the vivid scenes and emotional states you experienced as you watched them. Your subconscious does not differentiate between emotional states while watching shows and emotional states that arise from your own experiences. What you see on the screen adds to your subconscious belief patterns around pregnancy and birthing.

Reality TV shows that depict birth traumas and emergencies are popular because of the shock factor and the entertainment value experienced at a primal level, which affects the lower regions of the brain. Networks play these kinds of stories because normal healthy birth stories don't sell.

Fear and anxiety can take hold in women after hearing a traumatic birth story or watching a graphic birth scene as women are deeply affected emotionally by viewing other women's birth traumas.

In addition, the stress of feeling anxious or stressed while watching other people suffer has an immediate hormonal affect on your body and baby. The body produces stress hormones that can interfere with your baby's development and predispositions your baby for psychological issues after birth. When you experience unnecessary states of stress you tell your baby's body that the world they are about to enter is stressful. Instead you have an opportunity to prepare your baby for a universe that is supportive and loving.

The greatest obstacle blocking a painless childbirth is fear. The biggest fear is the fear of the unknown. You may have thought, *I don't know what is going to happen. I hear so much information and I want to be safe. I want my baby to be safe. I don't want to be in excruciating pain and I don't want to be vulnerable.*

Many women have no idea that painless childbirth is even a possibility. A significant percentage of women have claimed they have had a pleasurable birth or have experienced a blissful state with their natural childbirths.

What is a Recipe for a Healthy & Pain Free Childbirth?

- Empower yourself with positive birthing images and stories.

- Learn how normal and natural childbirth can be.

- Exercise during your pregnancy.

- Choose the best prenatal and birthing health care team for you.

- Educate your partner.

- Eliminate negative influences, such as TV, movies and stories from other women, that program you with fear and doubt.

- Use EFT to remove emotional blocks and fears around pregnancy and birthing.

- Learn abdominal breathing.

- Clear fears at the subconscious level using hypnotherapy.

- Cultivate a peaceful mindset.

- Use relaxation techniques.

- Learn about the realities of childbirth.

- Take a Hypnobabies or Hypnobirthing course.

Forget What You've Learned About Pregnancy From Hollywood

Birth is not only about making babies. Birth is about making mothers--strong, competent, capable mothers who trust themselves and know their inner strength.

~ Barbara Katz Rothman

When you watch TV or movies your conscious mind relaxes, but your subconscious is susceptible to suggestions and concepts. When you watch soap operas, dramas and movies your subconscious is taking in all the images and dialogue as though the information is fact. Since the entertainment industry generalizes, exaggerates, misrepresents and distorts pregnancy and the birthing process, women are collectively being programmed with myths and false information, which contributes to the way they feel and think about childbirth. In addition, it confuses pregnant women and expecting dads when they have experiences outside the limited range that TV-fantasyland provides.

Women in childbirth are mostly depicted by Hollywood as helpless, silly, insane with anger or constantly in danger. The entertainment industry has created a collective belief system around birthing that diminishes and hijacks a women's concept of pregnancy and childbirth. Some of the common stereotypes and false information that have been programmed into women include:

- Childbirth is not safe.
- Childbirth is always long and painful.
- Childbirth is complicated.
- Home birth or natural birth is not safe.
- A cesarean surgery is less painful and easier than vaginal birth.
- The water breaks and gushes out.
- Childbirth begins when the water breaks.
- Epidurals don't affect the baby.
- You have to give birth on your back.

If you'd like to watch birthing videos, instead watch videos that inspire you and fill you with joy. The belief you hold about birthing comes from all you have ever read, heard or seen about birthing. Empower yourself by watching confidence building and celebratory images of joyful, relaxed, peaceful women who are surrounded by supportive and loving family and friends, midwives, doulas and health care support. Women who actively move, change positions and even dance while in the birthing process often have easier and faster births.

You can find successful and peaceful natural childbirth videos on YouTube. You can also purchase the following recommended educational videos:

- Orgasmic Birth
- The Business of Being Born
- Birth Into Being
- Birth Day
- The Face of Birth

Enjoy the Healing Benefits of Nature

Every time my mother became pregnant, [my father] ... would announce to her that 'the glorious walks' must begin. These glorious walks consisted of him taking her to places of great beauty in the countryside and walking with her for about an hour each day so that she could absorb the splendor of the surroundings. His theory was that if the eye of a pregnant woman was constantly observing the beauty of nature, this beauty would somehow become transmitted to the mind of the unborn baby within her womb.

~ Ronald Dahl

Nature is a great place to meditate, reflect on life or experience profound states of gratitude. It is also a wonderful place to visit when you are feeling stressed and overwhelmed. Lying out on your lawn, exploring a cherished hiking trail or simply sitting by a lake can help rejuvenate, relax, inspire and heal you. Studies have shown that people who do not have regular access to a natural space often experience more stress than those who spend time in nature.

Aerosols From Trees

As you walk in nature, the trees, plants and flowers release healing properties into the air. Different trees have different healing compounds. For example, the black willow tree releases a type of antidepressant aerosol that is comforting and relieves loneliness. Pines produce an aerosol that has a healing and relaxing effect on the nervous system.[178]

Negative-Charged Ions

If you have ever been for a walk near the ocean or by a rushing stream, you may have noticed how relaxed and alive you feel. One of the reasons is that the air is filled with beneficial negatively charged ions that are produced from water molecules breaking apart as they hit the land. You can also get this affect when in a shower or with a small indoor fountain. However, the best way to get exposure to negative ions is to go outside. Plants and trees also give off negatively charged ions.

Researchers have found that seasonal depression[179] and chronic depression[180] can be successfully treated with exposure to negative ions. In other studies, negatively charged ions have been shown to reduce the physical effects of anxiety. Research suggests that negatively charged ions increase our ability to absorb and utilize oxygen, which benefits the brain, nervous system and all aspects of physical health.

Negatively charged ions are good for the health of your mind, as they promote alpha brainwaves and increase brainwave amplitude. The effect is a heightened sense of awareness combined with a calming influence. In studies on children with disabilities, exposure to negative ions showed remarkable improvements in their brain function.[181]

Some of the best places to explore include natural parks and treed areas, uninhabited land that is far from industry and cities and natural water sources such as coastal shorelines, lakes and waterfalls. Regardless of where you live, discover a place in nature that nourishes your body, mind and soul.

Avoid Air Pollution

For breath is life, and if you breathe well you will live long on earth.

~ *Sanskrit Proverb*

The quality of air you breathe is an essential element in the overall health of your baby. Prenatal exposure to air pollution from the burning of fossil fuels can negatively affect your baby's cognitive development. One study discovered that children exposed to high levels of hydrocarbons in utero scored lower on IQ tests when they reached the age of five, than children who were not exposed.[182] Other studies revealed that prenatal air pollution exposure triggers inflammation of the nervous system,[183] predisposes offspring to weight gain later in life,[184] increases anxiety, depression and behavioral problems[185] and affects lung development and lung health in offspring.[186]

Spend as much time in healthy environments with fresh indoor and outdoor air quality. When you can, walk in a forest, by the ocean or any area where nature offers the blessing of purifying the air for you.

Go for a Walk

Above all, do not lose your desire to walk. Every day I walk myself into a state of well-being and walk away from every illness. I have walked myself into my best thoughts, and I know of no thought so burdensome that one cannot walk away from it.

~ *Soren Kierkegaard*

While pregnant, daily walking is one of the best forms of exercise, as it is the easiest, cheapest and least impactful of all available exercise practices. No wonder it is one of the most popular activities during pregnancy. Combined with healthy nutrition, researchers have determined that daily walking of low or vigorous intensity is safe and beneficial to mom and baby.[187]

In addition, walking is a wonderful way to reduce stress and relax the body and mind. The movement of the muscles and joints improves circulation, increases the flow of energy and releases tension.

If you have the time, I recommend walking two times per day for 20 minutes each time. If walking is your only prenatal exercise, walk at least 20 minutes each day.

I find the best times to walk are early morning, late afternoon and at sunset. Early morning and late afternoon are great times to enjoy healthy sunshine without the harmful UVA and UVB rays. Early morning after the sun rises is a special time. The air is fresh, there is less pollution in the air and the birds are often singing. Walking with your partner near sunset is an excellent opportunity for bonding, sharing dreams and discussing issues. Make sure you get some kisses and eye gazing in along the way.

If you live in a colder or wetter climate, get outside anyway! Just throw on warm clothing and a good pair of footwear and enjoy the fresh air and exercise.

One of the best benefits of walking outdoors is the sensual interaction with the air, sun, sounds, smells and sights of nature. When I walk on my own, I take the opportunity to be really present with my experience. If thoughts or issues arise while walking, I may use some of the strategies I've shared in this book, like Emotional Freedom Technique, to clear emotional blocks or lingering issues that need attention. I always feel lighter, happier and more relaxed after I've gone for a walk.

Get Dirty

Gardening is how I relax.
It's another form of creating and playing with colors.

~ Oscar de la Renta

If you have the opportunity to garden, the engagement with nature while doing focused tasks can be one of the most relaxing and satisfying activities. Gardening reduces stress, promotes positive mood, decreases cortisol levels and research has found that gardening can even support relief from acute stress.[188]

Planting a seed and watching it grow nourishes the soul at a profound level. Cultivate a relationship with your garden, talk to it and send it your love. You may be surprised at how good it feels to co-create with nature and to nurture a garden space that ultimately nourishes your body, mind and soul.

If you don't have a garden space, buy a plant or two for your home. I love how my plants enliven my living space and turn it into an oasis. I've watched my plants grow from small little plants to their size today and I feel like they are part of the family. I love all of my plants, but one plant in particular was given to my husband and I for a wedding anniversary and holds a sweet spot in my heart.

Get Some Sunshine

Exposure to sunlight is one of the basic requirements for good health.

~ Tara Bianca

Sunshine nourishes you and helps grow your developing baby. The blessings of sunshine on the skin range from improving your complexion to balancing your hormones to promoting the absorption of calcium from the small intestine. Solar prana is also a source of life giving vital energy for your organs and helps to strengthen and revitalize your body.

Ultraviolet light acts as a natural antiseptic that can kill viruses, bacteria, mites, yeasts, fungi and mold. Getting some sun can help to clear up various skin conditions such as psoriasis, acne, eczema, athlete's foot and diaper rash.

Sunlight also stimulates your appetite and improves your digestion, elimination, metabolism and circulation. Having trouble sleeping at night? Exposure to natural light during the day increases your melatonin output at night, which enhances sleep and slows down the aging process. Sunlight increases the production of endorphins and serotonin in your brain leaving you feeling much better.

Sunlight is required to convert cholesterol into Vitamin D. There are Vitamin D receptors in almost every cell of the human body, demonstrating the importance of it as an essential part of maintaining balanced health. Vitamin D is required for the development of healthy bones and muscles. It also contributes to a reduction in inflammation in the body. Avoiding sunlight can contribute to vitamin D deficiency.

Those living in northern countries are aware of the effects of lack of sunshine on mental health during winter months. A lack of vitamin D can lead to seasonal affective disorder (SAD) with symptoms such as fatigue, sadness and, if severe enough, debilitating depression. SAD is most common in countries that are furthest from the equator and usually only occurs during the winter months when sunlight levels are low, although it can happen during the summer for those who use chemical sunscreen or who do not get outside enough.

You may find this surprising, although genes play a significant role in the final height of a person, research studies have found that prenatal sunlight is one of the most significant contributing factors for a newborn's height.189 Also, ultraviolet light B (UVB) exposure in the third trimester is related to increased bone density and mineral content in the child.190

Having a very fair complexion, I grew up avoiding the sun. My parents were overly cautious about my skin getting burnt. As a child, if I spent some time in the sun, I experienced extremely painful sunburns.

When I turned 30, I successfully transformed my relationship with the sun. Here are some key discoveries that have allowed me to safely soak up the sun to reap its beautiful benefits:

- **First**, I realized that the first exposures to the sun in the spring needed to be gradual.

- **Second**, and this was key, I found that the type of food I ate had a huge affect on whether I tanned or burned. Eating heavy cooked foods and processed junk foods contributed to burns. The more living, water rich raw foods I ate, the safer I seemed to be in the sun, especially with foods high in potassium and rich in vitamins and minerals. Essential fatty acids help restore skin elasticity and make your skin more burn resistant and regenerative. Also, it is important to drink plenty of water to hydrate the body.

- **Third**, I stopped wearing sunscreen. In the past, I seemed to burn even with the highest SPF sunscreens. There is evidence that most sunscreens are carcinogenic. Instead of wearing sunscreen, I learned from a wise woman in Costa Rica, that once you come out of the sun, cover your skin thinly with coconut oil or cold pressed olive oil mixed with a bit of water. I modified this advice by also lightly coating my skin with coconut oil mixed with a bit of water an hour before I go out into the sun.

- **Fourth**, I learned the importance of wearing a hat to protect the face, eyes and ears.

- **Fifth**, for the most part, I stayed out of the sun between 11am and 4pm. I limit myself to about 20 - 40 minutes at a time and make sure I give myself more time in the shade throughout the day. I especially love reclining on the grass in the full sun around 9am for some sunbathing.

It took one summer to transition my skin into sun loving and it was worth it! Not only does sunlight help fruit, vegetables and grains to grow and be healthy, sunlight helps humans to grow and be healthy, too. Enjoy a little sunshine today!

Enjoy Making Love

Making love is a sacred experience.

~ *Osho*

Unless your health care provider advises you otherwise, sex during pregnancy is safe for you and your baby. If you feel sexually aroused and are interested in being sexual, it is perfectly normal to have sex during pregnancy and it can be a wonderful way to bond with your partner. In fact, many women experience a burst of arousal during their second trimester. Their hormones get revved up and many of the side effects that may have left them feeling tired and nauseous in the first trimester have subsided. In addition, studies have shown that sexual interaction and physical affection improve mood and reduce stress for both men and women.

Here are a few guidelines for making love during your pregnancy:

1. *Be open with your partner.* Communicate your needs, preferences and true desires with your partner. The hormones associated with pregnancy may open up stronger passion and sensitivity. You and your partner may be surprised by the intensity of your sex drive, especially in the second trimester. Enjoy your heightened passion and impulses to deepen into intimacy with each other.

2. *Be true to you.* If you are not interested in sex, don't do it. Also make sure that your partner knows when something you used to like does not feel pleasurable. Being open about how your body's changes affect your sexual desires will help keep sexual play pleasurable for both of you. Since anxious thoughts about hurting the baby can

create stress for you and the baby, learn to let go of negative thoughts and feel relaxed about making love.

3. *Listen to your partner.* Your partner will have his own personal feelings about being sexual while you are pregnant. Take the time to listen to his fears and concerns. If either of you is not willing to have intercourse, explore new ways of pleasuring each other and connecting emotionally.

4. *Focus on touch.* Intercourse is just one of a number of forms of sexual contact. If you are in the mood to connect through caressing, touching, massaging or cuddling, communicate those needs as they arise. Remember to explore the needs and desires of your partner, as well.

5. *Make it a sacred experience.* Enjoy making love and give yourself over to the sacredness of connecting at the heart with your lover. Be willing to let go and surrender to the intimate interaction. Allow the pleasure of the experience to heal your body and connect you even stronger to your partner.

6. *Be creative.* Experiment with new positions to accommodate your expanding belly and changes to your body. If you are used to being the receptive force in your sexual explorations, experiment with being the more active, passionate and creative force.

7. *Listen to your body.* Be mindful, respectful and patient with your body. Allow it to guide you into what is comfortable.

If you are single, avoid having sex with strangers and whose sexual history is unknown. There are many diseases that can affect your baby's health and quality of life. While protection is a smart choice, using protection, such as a condom, is not a 100% safe guard for your baby.

Note: Contact your health care provider if you have concerns or if you experience unusual pain, spotting or contractions. Do not have intercourse if your membranes (bag of waters) have ruptured.

Encourage Loving Touch Between You & Your Partner

A single exposure of oxytocin can create a lifelong change in the brain.

~ Sue Carter, Chicago Psychiatric Institute

Loving touch is an essential need for humans young and old. Touch is the first sense to develop in the embryo with all other senses being derived from it.[191] It is one of the most powerful forms of communication and is the first language we learn. Without touch humans are more susceptible to stress, anxiety, depression and self-confidence issues.

Although loving touch can be used in conjunction with sexual touch, it is important to distinguish between loving and sexual touch. Women tend to understand the differences and often long for more non-sexual loving touch. Whereas men, although they enjoy non-sexual touch, often think of loving touch as a stepping stone to sex.

What is Loving Touch?

Loving touch is non-sexual and can include hugs, snuggles, cuddling, laying in each other's arms, holding hands, dancing, massage, gentle touch and body work. One of the benefits to loving touch is the release of oxytocin, which immediately reverses our body's response to stress, assists in the healing of previous relationships and primes the brain to be less reactive to stress in the future.

The healing power of loving touch is extraordinary. Loving touch fosters love and respect, contributes to over all emotional and psychological health, stimulates vital physiological systems, improves circulation and general well-being, increases relaxation, reduces stress and aids in healing. It also develops intimacy, closeness, meaningful memories, bonding and trust.

Romance Your Partner

A successful marriage requires falling in love many times,
always with the same person.

~ Mignon McLaughlin

Take responsibility for cultivating intimacy between you and your partner by creating opportunities for playful, romantic interactions each and every day. Hold each other in loving embraces, practice gazing into each other's eyes and enjoy holding hands when walking together.

As a couple, it is also important to plan one night a week to go on a date or to stay in with the purpose of connecting at the heart. While the occasional movie can be a nice way to snuggle up together, it does not cultivate intimacy.

207

If you choose to go to see a film, plan to have dinner before or to go for an after movie herbal tea or smoothie. Although favorite restaurants and activities are comfortable and enduring, if you are adventurous try new activities or venues to create new experiences for you to share together. Examples include taking a class together, going to a new restaurant, snuggling at an art gallery, walking in an area you've never explored before or just watching the sun set.

If you find that it is difficult to get out, have a romantic evening at home. You don't need to go out to bond with your partner. Cook a nice meal together, have breakfast in bed, play a fun board game or enjoy spending time connecting in more intimate ways. If you have children, plan your romantic evening to begin after the kids go to bed or arrange for them to stay with family or friends. Spending quality time together, cultivates intimacy, which helps reduce stress.

In addition to setting aside time to connect with your sweetheart, romance your partner by noticing the good and appreciating what your partner is doing to care for you and support you. Assume the best about your partner and express your gratitude for being cared for, loved, protected and cherished. Let your partner know how much you love them by your actions, words and touch.

Wear Comfortable Clothing & Footwear

A woman is never sexier than when she is comfortable in her clothes.

~ *Vera Wang*

Feeling comfortable in your clothes and shoes is a high priority while pregnant. During pregnancy there are many sensations and changes clamoring for attention. Wearing tight or uncomfortable clothing and shoes during pregnancy can result in irritation, leading to stress.

Comfort is great, but it does not have to mean that you throw style out the window. Clothing is a huge part of our identity and can be a factor in how good we feel. Today, many maternity lines provide cutting edge style while still maintaining the comfort level that leaves women feeling beautiful. With that in mind, it is important to remember a few things about purchasing clothes that are comfortable for you throughout your pregnancy.

1. *Plan ahead if you are on a budget.* Remember that your body is constantly changing throughout your pregnancy. Make sure that you purchase clothes that will still be comfortable during the last few weeks of your pregnancy.

2. *Choose fabrics that are natural.* Not only are synthetics made from chemicals, they also have a tendency to not allow your skin to breathe as well as natural fabrics, such as cotton. Most manufacturers add chemicals, such as formaldehyde, to prevent mildew growth during oversees shipping. Make sure you wash your new clothes before wearing them. Whenever possible, purchase organically produced clothing.

3. *Choose shoes that offer support but are easy to get on or off.* Avoid flip-flops, which have been linked to knee and back damage and can cause injuries. For comfort and safety avoid high heels.

Start a New Hobby

When your hobbies get in the way of your work - that's OK;

but when your hobbies get in the way of themselves... well.

~ *Steve Martin*

If you feel stressed, why not start a new hobby or fun activity. Enjoying a new activity assists the mind to focus on a task, relax and let go of its need to think about stressful thoughts. In addition, having a hobby stimulates creativity, offers scheduled time for relaxation, creates social opportunities and cultivates new skills. Mental stimulation through learning a new hobby improves brain functioning, improves mood and creates new neural pathways.

Here are some pregnancy friendly hobbies to consider:

- ✓ Join a book club.
- ✓ Take a photography or art class.
- ✓ Scrapbook, journal, write poetry or short stories.
- ✓ Explore crafting, sewing, embroidery or knitting.
- ✓ Learn to play the piano or an instrument.

✓ Do some beading or jewelry making.

✓ Enjoy gardening.

✓ Take a nutrition course.

✓ Learn to make healthy cultured foods like yogurt, kefir and sauerkraut.

Rest When You Can

Activity and rest are two vital aspects of life. To find a balance in them is a skill in itself. Wisdom is knowing when to have rest, when to have activity, and how much of each to have. Finding them in each other - activity in rest and rest in activity - is the ultimate freedom.

~ Sri Sri Ravi Shankar, Celebrating Silence: Excerpts from Five Years of Weekly Knowledge 1995-2000

As your pregnancy progresses, your body will require more rest as resources are needed for the development of the baby. One of the most nourishing things you can do for you and your baby is to take the time to rest or nap throughout the day. When you rest, you allow your body to recharge, which frees up energy to nourish the baby.

Listen to your body. Your pregnancy is only a short amount of time in the spectrum of your life, so give yourself permission to rest to avoid health complications and getting over-exhausted. Rest is especially essential in the last two months. Take every opportunity to rest and nap in preparation for birthing your baby. If napping interferes with your nighttime sleep, resting can still help reenergize your body and mind.

Get Enough Sleep

Sleep is the best meditation.

~ *Dalai Lama*

In addition to air, water and food, sleep is just one of those things that you need to live. With the exception of rare cases, the body can only go for a few days without sleep before the brain begins to be impaired. Sufficient sleep is essential to proper brain functioning and health. Without sleep mental performance wanes, hormones show signs of disruption, memory loss becomes apparent and your risk for diabetes[192] and high blood pressure increases.

Sleep deprivation impairs the healing process. Your body and mind suffer from lack of sleep and will show it through signs of stress. As well, sleeping issues are almost always involved in psychiatric and mental disorders such as depression, anxiety, Alzheimer's disease and schizophrenia. The variance of symptoms change depending on the amount of sleep a person experiences.

Why You Might Have Trouble Sleeping?

Sleep and wakefulness come in waves. If you find yourself feeling tired at night, go to bed. When you push through and stay awake, you may miss a window of opportunity for natural sleep. I know many people who eat when they feel slightly tired at night, because they think it will energize them. The stimulating effect is a false sense of energy, which works against the body's natural rhythm to sleep. I suggest not eating three hours before bedtime, as it stimulates and activates the body to wake up.

Stress is a huge influencing factor on a person's ability to sleep. When the mind is overactive, it can keep you up at night. Thinking about the next day's activities or dwelling on an issue contributes to stress and anxiety. Psychological stress, such as anxiety and depression, affects the brain-body chemistry by depleting neurotransmitters, which contributes to difficulty sleeping and insomnia. If there is a known underlying event or emotional conflict, do your best to resolve the issue. Ultimately, seek professional help for all unmanageable or long-term issues of depression.

Neurotransmitter depletion can also be caused by nutritional stress and physiological stress such as a nutrient deficient diet, eating junk food, medications such as SSRIs, over consumption of chocolate and other stimulants, sensory overload of sounds, lights and fast movement, chronic pain, over work, Candida, irritable bowel disorder (IBS), food allergies and food sensitivities. Deficiency in GABA (an essential neurotransmitter for inducing sleep, motor control, vision and the regulation of anxiety) may also show up with symptoms such as IBS, constipation, blurred vision, irritability, allergies, anxiousness, dizziness and mood disorders.

Although GABA cannot be obtained directly from your diet, precursors to GABA and other neurotransmitters like Vitamin B-6, L-theanine and L-glutamine can be obtained from food. Sources of Vitamin B-6 are potatoes, broccoli, spinach, bell peppers, kale, summer squash, shiitake mushrooms, avocado, sunflower seeds, oranges, bananas and animal protein. Foods rich in L-theanine include spinach and whole grains. Great sources of L-glutamine can be found in cabbage, beans, beets, almonds, lentils, dairy products, animal protein and spinach.

Insomnia and difficulty sleeping, as well as restless legs, anxiety, depression, anger and hyper-emotionality can also result from chronic magnesium deficiency. Natural sources of magnesium include foods high in chlorophyll such as dark, leafy greens and green vegetables, as well as unrefined, whole grains, peas, nuts and seeds. Restless legs may also be a result of calcium or iron deficiency.

Side Effects of Sleeping Pills

Long-term use of sleeping pills creates a drugged effect rather than a nourishing, satisfying and restful sleep. Agitation and wakefulness can occur as a result of chemical withdrawal when a person suddenly stops using sleeping pills. As the FDA has not approved any medication safe for a fetus, sleeping pills are not recommended. In addition, new research shows that sleeping pills increase your risk of dying.[193]

Sleep Issues During Pregnancy

Sufficient sleep is imperative while you are pregnant, as your quality and quantity of sleep affects not only you but also your baby. During pregnancy your sleep needs will increase and your sleep patterns may change. Most expecting moms experience some form of alterations to their sleep at some point during their pregnancy. Morning sickness, hormonal changes, restless legs, frequent urination and expansion of your belly during late pregnancy can all contribute to a variety of sleep issues.

Although most recommendations for sleep fall along the general rule of eight hours for adults, many people do better with seven to nine hours. When you are pregnant, the key is to listen to your body. If you need 10 or 12 hours, go to bed early or sleep in late.

If you've familiarized yourself with EFT (review the section called "Use Emotional Freedom Technique"), you can tap with any truthful set up phrase on the **Karate Chop Point** around difficulty sleeping. Some phrases might include:

- Even though I am tired, but I'm having difficulty falling asleep, I fully and completely love and accept myself.
- Even though I'm feeling frustrated because I can't sleep, I fully and completely love and accept myself.
- Even though I am worried I'll just lie awake if I go to bed, I am open to see what happens.

The other tapping points may include phrases like the following:

Top of the Head: I feel tense.

Eyebrow: I feel tired.

Side of the Eye: And I'm afraid I won't be able to fall asleep.

Under the Eye: Even though I have this fear and frustration…

Chin: I can lie down and rest.

Collarbone: And love and accept myself…

Under the Arm: Even though a part of me resists sleep.

Top of the Head: I can allow myself to sleep deeply,

Eyebrow: in this comfortable bed.

Side of the Eye: It's okay to fall asleep.

Under the Eye: I can let go,

Chin: and rest into these pillows,

Collarbone: release all the tension,

Under the Arm: and feel safe.

Inhale a deep breath through your nose and exhale a Haaaah sound out loud. Repeat this two more times.

Insomnia

Researchers have observed that chronic stress contributes to chronic insomnia.[194] If you experience insomnia during your pregnancy, during the day ensure that you rest, nap, walk and eat a balanced, healthy diet. If you develop persistent sleep issues or insomnia, see your health care professional for additional advice.

Cultivate Healthy Sleep Habits

- Avoid alcohol and caffeine.

- Don't eat or drink within 2-3 hours of going to bed. However, during pregnancy you most likely will need to drink water and possibly eat something if you feel hungry. If you eat something, choose easily digestible, nutritional whole foods. Avoid full meals, dairy and wheat based foods late at night.

- After dinner, write out any tasks that need to be completed the next day or later that week to clear them from your mind.

- Give yourself at least 30 minutes each night before bedtime to relax and prepare for sleep.

- Avoid stimulating activities prior to bed, such as watching TV, working, cleaning or being on the computer, iPod or other electrical devices.

- Begin turning off lights around the house or dimming lights two hours before bedtime.

- Go to bed and wake up at the same time seven days a week, including weekends.

- Go to bed at least one hour before midnight. When you go to bed late, you risk missing the natural wave of sleep readiness your body feels. Go to bed even earlier if you need it. You are growing a baby, which takes a lot of energy.

- Sleep in a darkened, cool room.

- Keep your bedroom reserved for sleep only. Remove all unnecessary electronics. Remove adapters or make sure they are over four feet from your body.

- Spend some time connecting with your partner and your baby before sleep.

- If your partner snores, use earplugs or in severe cases establish separate beds for sleeping.

- Do some relaxed, easy, deep belly breathing as you are lying in bed. If you find your mind wandering, just bring yourself back to the breath in the body.

Listen To Some Inspirational, Relaxing or Motivating Music

Beautiful music is the art of the prophets that can calm the agitations of the soul;
it is one of the most magnificent and delightful presents God has given us.

~ *Martin Luther*

Music moves the soul and vibrates the cells. It frees the mind and opens the heart. We all have experienced the magic of music and the significant role it has played in our lives. When a particular song plays, it can transport you back to that moment stirring up emotions as though you are there again.

The type of music you listen to is important as it influences your mood and energy. Studies have found that the effects of classical and meditative music improve cardiovascular and respiratory health more than other types of music. On the other hand, heavy metal, techno or very fast tempo music can contribute to stress.

Music is often very relaxing and can induce the conscious mind into a more receptive state. The subconscious mind is forever in an open state and has no filter and takes everything on as though it is reality. Song lyrics are like seeds that get planted in the garden of your mind. They will grow into belief systems and energetic patterns that show up in your life. That is why it is important to ensure that the lyrics within the songs you listen to are uplifting, positive and support the state of mind you would like to cultivate. Be intentional with your music choices. Play your favorites and explore music that nourishes, inspires and relaxes you.

Maternal Benefits of Music

Music therapy or daily exposure to relaxing music has demonstrated a reduction of maternal stress, anxiety and depression in expecting women.[195] In general, benefits attributed to listening to classical and meditation music include the reduction of sleep problems, an increase in sleep quality and a reduction of depressive symptoms, anxiety, blood pressure, heart rates, respiratory rates and sympathetic nervous system activity.[196]

Music for Mom Influences Baby, Too

Maternal music exposure has proven beneficial to neonatal behavior and health. Listening to relaxing music for a minimum of 30 minutes per day has an affect on reducing maternal stress and anxiety.[197] Infants of mothers who were exposed to 50 minutes of relaxing music every evening during pregnancy also performed better on assessments measuring orientation, habituation and motor performance.[198] Anytime a mom's stress is reduced, the effect will be beneficial on the developing baby.

Music for Baby

The healthy development of your baby's brain is essential. Studies have shown that music played during pregnancy increases the neuron development in the hippocampus and enhances spatial learning ability of animal[199] [200] and human offspring. In the last trimester, prenatal exposure to music influences auditory functional development of the fetus.[201] Fetuses can easily hear music played at the same volume as normal conversations. Avoid putting speakers against your belly as it can over stimulate the developing auditory system or may interfere with your baby's sleep-wake cycle.

Exercise, But Don't Over Do Physical Activity

I have to exercise in the morning before my brain figures out what I'm doing.

~ Marsha Doble

US National Guidelines recommend that healthy pregnant women exercise for 30 minutes or more per day because of the many prenatal and postnatal benefits it provides both you and your baby.

Prenatal Benefits

There are many benefits to exercising when pregnant including a healthier prenatal experience and easier child birthing. Researchers have found that expecting women who exercised in the first 20 weeks of pregnancy experienced a significant reduction in risk for gestational diabetes[202] and pre-eclampsia.[203] [204] Low intensity exercises such as stretching,[205] yoga and tai chi[206] produce physiological benefits including reduced stress and lowered blood pressure. Prenatal exercise:

✓ Relieves tension and stress.

✓ Increases energy and improves mood.

✓ Improves muscular strength, which enhances your ability to carry your growing baby.

✓ Reduces or eliminates pregnancy discomfort.

✓ Helps prevent pre-eclampsia.

✓ Reduces or prevents the risk of complications during and after the birthing process.

- ✓ Lowers the risk of birth defects, developmental issues and health complications in the baby.

- ✓ Supports your baby's neurological and physical development.

- ✓ Contributes to a healthy self-esteem.

- ✓ Helps to strengthen and tone your pelvic floor.

- ✓ Helps to minimize stretch marks.

- ✓ Helps to circulate energy throughout the body.

- ✓ Improves posture.

- ✓ Improves your stamina for birthing.

Although there are many benefits to exercising when pregnant, avoid over exercising as it may contribute to overheating, ketosis, exhaustion, physical stress to your body and stress on the baby. It is a good idea to limit exercising to an hour per exercise period and no more than 10 hours per week. It is also important to listen to your body's signs for rest, replenishment of water, electrolytes and nourishment.

Some fitness activities may need to be modified during your pregnancy, so it is a good idea to join prenatal versions of activities. Some of these include aerobics, aquafit, dance, yoga or Pilates.

Fitness activities and sports to avoid during pregnancy include contact sports, high altitude activities and risk related activities such as boxing, basketball, hockey, rugby, soccer, diving, scuba diving, whitewater rafting, gymnastics, horseback riding, ice skating, rollerblading, downhill skiing, snow boarding, hang gliding, parachuting, base jumping, bungee jumping, rock climbing and mountain climbing.

If you are beginning a new fitness regime after conceiving or you are uncertain about how much exercise is best suited to your pregnancy, listen to your body and consult with your health care provider.

Best Types of Exercise:

If you are not the exercising type, at least walk or swim for 20 minutes each day. If you enjoy exercise, some of the best activities to do while pregnant include:

- ✓ Walking, jogging or hiking
- ✓ Pilates or yoga
- ✓ Dancing or low impact aerobics
- ✓ Tai chi or chi kung
- ✓ Weight training
- ✓ Bicycling or spinning
- ✓ Cross country skiing or skiing machine
- ✓ Aquafit, swimming or snorkeling
- ✓ Kegel pelvic floor exercises

Dance

I see dance being used as communication between body and soul,
to express what is too deep to find for words.

~ Ruth St. Denis

Dancing while pregnant is a delicious celebration of beauty, strength, power and freedom. It is also a fun non-impact form of exercise to keep you feeling energized and your body flexible and strong. You can dance in the privacy of your own home anytime by just putting on some motivating music and moving your body as you feel inspired. Inspirational dance can allow you to express yourself from the depths of your soul. You can even make it a dance dedicated to the love you feel for your baby!

If you're not sure how to get into the groove, purchase a prenatal instructional dance DVD. If you feel drawn to dance with other expecting moms, attend a local prenatal dance class in your area. Belly dancing is a favorite of many expecting women.

Birthing moms have also been known to use dancing during the birthing process to relieve tension, disperse pain and to ease fetal movement in the second stage of birthing. Dancing with your partner is an intimate way to bond during your childbirth. Visit YouTube for inspirational videos of women dancing during childbirth. The benefits of prenatal dancing include:

- Relaxing the body
- Promoting health posture
- Relieving lower back pain
- Reducing mental and physical stress

- Strengthening pelvic and abdominal muscles
- Lowering blood pressure

Suggestions for Safe Dancing

While dancing, avoid jerky or high impact movement that may increase your risk of injury. Remember to stay hydrated. Listen to your body and be mindful as your centre of gravity changes as your baby grows. Avoid deep bends, over stretching or movements that cause pain or discomfort. Seek your health care provider's advice before starting any exercise program.

Join a Prenatal Yoga Class

You cannot do yoga. Yoga is your natural state. What you can do are yoga exercises, which may reveal to you where you are resisting your natural state.

~ Sharon Gannon

Yoga is a great way to reduce stress and relieve tension during your pregnancy. Scheduling in a weekly prenatal yoga class is also a wonderful way to set aside some relaxing time for you. Listening to your body is essential any time you do yoga, but it is especially imperative when you are pregnant. Don't push yourself if you are feeling pain, light-headedness or discomfort. Avoid Bikram or hot yoga classes, as overheating can cause stress to your baby.

I highly recommend that even advanced yoginis take prenatal yoga classes rather than regular classes as the instructor is trained to present modified poses, as well as provide support and instruction tailored to the pregnant body.

224

Benefits of Prenatal Yoga

Prenatal yoga is known to help women remain limber and flexible, build strength, improve focus and concentration, increase energy, relieve tension, reduce stress and anxiety, improve circulation, establish healthy breathing techniques and meet other expecting moms.

Get a Massage

Take care of your body.
It's the only place you have to live.

~ Jim Rohn

As your pregnancy progresses, you may begin to feel the pressures and pains that come with additional weight, hormones and changes to your overall structural alignment. Prenatal massage is a great way to assist you to relax, alleviate muscle pain and relieve some of the tension your body is carrying. It is helpful for improving circulation and muscle tone in your body and blood flow to the baby. Prenatal massage also relieves stress and improves mood by boosting levels of serotonin and endorphins, which are the body's natural mood regulators and painkillers.

Depending on how many months along you are in your pregnancy, prenatal massage can have some important differences than regular massage. Ensure that your practitioner is certified or trained in prenatal massage and they have the equipment to support your body. Avoid massages in spas where the staff tend not to have prenatal massage experience. During a high-risk pregnancy, first consult with your prenatal health care provider.

Pregnancy massage from your partner is also a great way for you to connect and build intimacy together. Whole body massages are great, but a localized massage to the forehead or hands can be just the trick to melt away the tension. Even a three to five minute foot massage can produce delicious relaxation.

Take a Mini Holiday

For fast-acting relief try slowing down.

~ Lily Tomlin

A great way to reduce stress and to relax is to go on a mini holiday to a nearby bed and breakfast for the weekend. Spending time away from your normal distractions of phone, computer, household chores and making meals gives the mind a break. The brain also likes to experience new things and releases dopamine during pleasurable experiences. Dopamine helps to reduce stress, increase creativity, stimulate new connections, improve memory and sharpen mental focus.

Be sure to make your getaway a romantic one. A romantic getaway offers couples a refreshing change of pace and devoted time with each other. Take walks arm in arm, cuddle in bed and gaze lovingly into each other's eyes. Be sure to pack romantic music and massage oil. Most of all enjoy the time you spend together. Make a rule to leave household issues at home. Take the opportunity to relax and get to know each other all over again. You'd be surprised how rejuvenating and inspiring a little getaway can be.

Be Grateful

There are only two ways to live your life.
One is as though nothing is a miracle.
The other is as if everything is.

~ *Albert Einstein*

There is so much unbelievable beauty in this world. There has never been, nor will there ever be two days alike. Enjoy the blessings of how each moment unfolds before your very eyes. Opportunities for delight and gratitude abound.

Begin with you; you are a miracle of life. Trillions of cells in your body dance around, working on your behalf. Every aspect of your body, mind and energy system is integrated and complex, yet efficient and intelligent in its design. Your body-mind-energy triad performs 24/7 with little to no direction or input from you. Your body is carrying a divine process of creation. It can't help but inform you and change you for the rest of your life. You are a garden, the soil for the little sprout within you. The sun shines upon you, the birds sing for you and your partner and family were all designed to take this journey with you. The universe exists for you and you for it.

If you find it difficult to feel grateful, it may be because you think that life should be different than it is. Judgment makes it impossible to experience gratitude. Gratitude naturally arises when you let go of the need to change yourself, others and the world.

Simple & Powerful Gratitude Practices
* Each time you drink a glass of water or eat food, say 'thank you.'

- At the end of every day, write in a journal five things for which are you are most grateful from your day.

- Imagine all the things in the universe that had to align so that you are here in this moment.

- Take time to reflect upon the people and miracles that have blessed in your life.

Practice Loving-Kindness

You yourself, as much as anybody in the entire universe,
deserve your love and affection.

~ Buddha

Loving-kindness is essential for a peaceful heart. It is a state of love and compassion that can be beautifully cultivated within your being. It begins with generating loving-kindness for yourself, then towards family, friends, strangers, enemies and all sentient beings. It allows for the deeply beautiful blessing of an opening heart that is free of sadness, anger and bitterness.

Benefits of loving-kindness include personal relaxation, peace, harmony, safety, friendliness, stress prevention, stress reduction, improved quality of sleep and releasing toxic emotions. There are many techniques that can be used to cultivate feelings of loving-kindness.

I was first introduced to a loving-kindness technique in university. I had been suffering from stress from an excessive workload and a lack of sleep. A wise man shared with me the following simple phrases to repeat every evening before I go to bed and any time I feel anxious or angry with myself or someone else:

- May I have physical happiness, may I have mental happiness, may I be at peace, may I be well.
- May my family have physical happiness, may they have mental happiness, may they be at peace, may they be well.
- May my friends have physical happiness, may they have mental happiness, may they be at peace, may they be well.
- May my community have physical happiness, may they have mental happiness, may they be at peace, may they be well.
- May everyone in the world have physical happiness, may they have mental happiness, may they be at peace, may they be well.

It transformed my anxious mind to one of relative peace for a young university student. I slept much better and my mind quieted down and released anxiety.

Later, I learned another loving-kindness technique at a Buddhist monastery that I refer to as *Planting Seeds of Loving-Kindness*. In this meditation, start by sitting in a comfortable position, either in a chair or on a cushion. I also do this before falling asleep in a lying down position. Begin breathing slowly and deeply, in and out, through the nose. Fill your abdomen with air as you inhale and slowly release the air as you exhale. Concentrate fully on your breathing. If thoughts arise, simply let them fade away and return your attention to the breath moving in and out of your belly. Continue with breathing until you feel relaxed.

Once your body and mind feel very relaxed, start to visualize the loving-kindness seeds as seeds you plant in your heart center. The seeds can be for loving-kindness flowers of any color that will blossom there once they are nurtured. I like to visualize purple flowers, but any color will do. Begin by repeating the phrase with your inner voice, *"May I be healthy, may I be joyful, may I be peaceful,"* over and over again. As you repeat the mantra, simultaneously see the seeds in your heart being watered and watch the flowers growing and blossoming before your inner eye. As your flowers grow, smile upon them with joy. You can offer the mantra and flowers over to benefit another person. Simply say, *"May my mother (or my neighbor) be healthy, may they joyful, may they be peaceful."*

Loving-kindness can be practiced almost anywhere: when you are stuck in traffic, on a plane, in a train, on a bus, as you sit in a park, at home or in the office. As you practice this meditation you will notice a change in your state of being and people around you will notice, too.

All that we are is the result of what we have thought.
The mind is everything. What we think we become.
~ Buddha

Practice Forgiveness

Peace begins with me, and no one else.

~ Dr. Ihaleakala Hew Len

When we hold unforgiveness in the heart toward our self or others we hold a wounding within us that affects our physical, mental and emotional health. We cannot undo the past, but we have the power to forgive and make amends.

Forgiveness requires courage to surrender the hurt in our heart and the ideas of wrongness in our mind. When we find that courage to release the sadness, anger and negativity, we allow for a new understanding and healing to emerge.

Forgiveness happens inside of you. Forgiveness doesn't mean that we forget or excuse another's behavior. Nor does it mean that we reunite with a person that has harmed us. The alternative of forgiveness is the perpetuation of denial, vengeance and anger. We have all done things wrong in the past and may have even broken someone's trust. So in forgiving others, we allow for ourselves to be forgiven and vice versa. Forgiveness of oneself and others provides an opportunity for growth and learning within the person doing the forgiving.

One of the most helpful and profound forgiveness practices I have come across is an ancient Hawaiian practice of reconciliation and forgiveness called Ho'oponopono (pronounced ho-o-pono-pono). Ho'oponopono means to make right and is defined in the Hawaiian Dictionary as "mental cleansing: family conferences in which relationships were set right through prayer, discussion, confession, repentance, and mutual restitution and forgiveness." [207]

Ho'oponopono Practice:

Dear _(name of person)_

I love you.

I am sorry for _____. (You can also add: I am sorry for any harm I have caused you in this lifetime or any other lifetime.)

Please forgive me.

Thank you. Thank you. Thank you.

The practice begins with connecting with the person at a heart level. Next, you take responsibility for whatever harm you've caused them. Then you ask for forgiveness. Saying thank you is an expression of gratitude for having the opportunity to learn and make things right. Remember to breathe deeply throughout this practice.

A deeper level of Ho'oponopono is based on the principle of 100% responsibility, **taking responsibility for everyone's actions, not only for one's own**. If one would take complete responsibility for one's life, then everything one sees, hears, tastes, touches or in any way experiences would be one's responsibility because it is in one's life. The problem and solution would not be with our external reality, it would be with ourselves. To change our reality, we would have to change ourselves. This does not have anything to do with feeling guilty. Instead it is a powerful reminder to return back to your true state free of suffering. In the words of the Buddha: To understand everything is to forgive everything.

Let Go of the Need to Be Superwoman

*Even when I'm a mess, I still put on a vest, With an S
on my chest, Oh yes, I'm a Superwoman.*

~ *Alicia Keys, Superwoman*

I'll be short and sweet with this one. Take care of yourself by letting go of the need to get involved in everything and to do it all. Doing it all is overrated. Get back to the basics – take care of your basic needs like resting, eating well and having fun. Listen to your body and ask for help when you need it!

Ask for Help

Asking is the beginning of receiving. Make sure you don't go to the ocean with a teaspoon. At least take a bucket so the kids won't laugh at you.

~ Jim Rohn

One of the most challenging strategies for some women to learn is to ask for help. In general, women have been the main caretakers of relationships and families, assisting and anticipating where they can help out next. However, they tend to take care of their needs last. Sometimes we need another set of ears or hands to assist us to resolve an issue. That assistance may be a friend, spouse, family member, neighbor, pastor, health care practitioner or even a stranger if necessary.

Whether you are experiencing emotional challenges, hormonal ups and downs, physical pain or need help to physically do things while you are pregnant, ask for help as soon as you recognize that you need it. Waiting until things get acutely stressful or require emergency intervention is often more difficult to resolve and the stress can contribute to premature birth or mental and physical developmental complications for your baby.

Women are great at getting things done. However, they can be impatient when they work on a task they are determined complete. Too many women lift heavy items, climb up on chairs or bend beyond their means instead of waiting for their partner or someone else to assist them.

A women's ability to safely lift a heavy load decreases in late pregnancy due to hormonal influences softening the connective tissue, ligaments and tendons. In some cases, lifting heavy items can even strain the abdominal area creating stress on the uterus and potentially doing damage to the placenta.

When pregnant even a slight injury can become annoying, stressful and problematic. Avoid lifting heavy items or bending beyond your means. Accidents and injuries can happen when we go beyond our limits, so wait for assistance. If you happen to be without your partner at a store, ask for help from a store employee to carry heavy items to your vehicle.

Hire a House Cleaner

My idea of housework is to sweep the room with a glance.

~ Erma Bombeck

Studies have shown that stress can often be linked to our environment. Having a messy house can often trigger stress in many ways. In addition, having to clean the house can be overwhelming when you add it to the list of your other responsibilities. During your pregnancy, it is important to delegate tasks, such as housecleaning, to others so you can maintain a healthy balance in your life. Share tasks with your partner or even children if they are old enough.

If you can afford it, consider hiring a weekly house cleaner to take care of the larger tasks to lessen your load. When you hire a house cleaner, decide whether you would want a single person or whether you would like to hire a service. Usually, a service is less expensive but you may not always get the same person. Regardless, take the time to check around with people you know to find out if there are any good house cleaners in your area.

Remember to follow these guidelines for hiring:

1. **Contact and interview multiple house cleaners.**

2. **Interview your candidates.** Take the time to interview each house cleaner to ensure which one is the best fit for you and your cleaning needs. Trust your instincts.

3. **Ensure they are bondable.** Always make sure that the people you hire are bondable with an up to date police check. Many times, house cleaners will come into your home when you are away so you want to make sure you can trust them.

4. **Ask for three references.** Ask for references and then check them to ensure they are valid.

Remember, a house cleaner is there to assist you. If you feel more stressed after employing a cleaner, then find someone who better suits your needs.

Set Some Limits

Half of the troubles of this life can be traced to saying yes too quickly and not saying no soon enough.

~ *Josh Billings*

During your pregnancy, setting limits should become an important part of maintaining the health of both you and your baby. You may believe you can do everything, but remind yourself that there are only so many hours in a day. To set boundaries, there are few guidelines that you can follow:

- **Become self-aware.** It is important to be aware of your own physical, mental and emotional limits. Also, be realistic about the available time you have for helping others, especially as you transition through pregnancy into motherhood.

- **Say "no."** Learn how to say "no" and decline offers. Setting limits can be difficult initially, but as you become more confident with your boundaries, you will find that your stress level reduces and you are much happier.

- **Communicate your limits in clear and respectful ways.** Express your needs, worries, feelings, concerns and opinions in ways that honor you and the other person.

- **Respect other people's boundaries.** It is just as important to respect other people's boundaries.

- **Welcome help.** If you are blessed with the gift of friends and family offering to help you, with gratitude, just say yes!

- **Ask for help.** When you need help, ask for it.

- **Be kind to yourself.** Setting limits for yourself in relationship to work and your personal life is a gift of kindness to you during your pregnancy.

- **Drop all guilt.** Let go of any need to mentally punish yourself when you need to cut back on work or personal activities. You are pregnant, which means your resources need to go to developing a growing baby. Instead, tell yourself what a great job you are doing when you take care of your needs by setting boundaries.

Give Yourself Permission to Relax

No matter how much pressure you feel at work, if you could find ways to relax
for at least five minutes every hour, you'd be more productive.

~ *Dr. Joyce Brothers*

Many women tend to find something to do every waking minute of the day. The persistent movement from one activity to another can be stressful when it is done in a frantic, "there's not enough hours in a day" kind of way. Exhaustion and stress show up in the busyness of the mind and in the tension of the body. This contributes to chemical and physical imbalances in the body that affect not only you but also your baby. Furthermore, you are chemically and energetically training your baby how to move through the world.

Create a Relaxation Schedule

By having a relaxation schedule, stress becomes a lot easier to manage. Give yourself permission to meet your own basic needs to enjoy a break. Learn to integrate a period of rest after significant tasks. Also, take 5-10 minutes every 50 minutes to get up and move around regardless if you are done a task or not.

If you need a more disciplined approach, schedule designated relaxation times throughout your day. Lunchtime is a great time to relax. Take your lunch to a park or a quiet area and enjoy every bite of your food. Schedule a walk in the park, a meditation/breathing exercise or a yoga class.

Relaxation Strategies

- Find inspiring locations to take your breaks where you can actually relax.

- If at any time you truly don't have time for a break, learn to relax while you do a task. The best way to accomplish this is to BREATHE and be as fully present as you can be.

- Finding joy in a task can also be a way to experience relaxation. I find doing the dishes very satisfying. The feeling of my hands in warm water and the sense of simple accomplishment each time I wash and rinse a dish is relaxing.

- Give yourself a small break from mental worry by visualizing your worries or stresses being tied to a hot air balloon and going up into the sky. You can also make time to do a five-minute holiday visualization of you relaxing on a beach.

Make a commitment to creating a healthy habit of relaxation. Relaxing is an investment in your health and in the health of your child.

Turn Out the Lights

We are the music makers, and we are the dreamers of dreams.

~ Arthur O'Shaughnessy

Have you ever felt overwhelmed by everything that is happening around you: the way your brain and body feel, the hum of the lights, the sound of the television or the radio, the constant whirl of computers, telephones or the multitude of other things that can overwhelm the senses? All of that

238

stimulation can compound and contribute to stress, especially when you are pregnant.

Take a mini blackout break from all the stimulation by turning off all sources of noise, going to your bedroom, turning off the lights (or covering your eyes) and laying down. Then close your eyes and just breathe. Continue to bring in the breath into your belly and feel your body. If your mind wanders a little, guide it into daydreams of open fields of flowers or a mountain stream. Envision yourself taking in the nourishment of the peace and tranquility.

Establish Balance in Your Weekly Schedule

Happiness is not a matter of intensity but of balance, order, rhythm and harmony.

~ Thomas Merton

We all need a balance of play, work, learning, exercise, nutrition, reflection and sleep, as well as time with others and time to ourselves. One of the first steps in establishing balance is to set a schedule that ensures it. The key is to have a base schedule that allows you to meet all your needs while at the same time remaining flexible to what life brings your way.

Go to bed and wake up at the same time each day, eat at the same times, schedule times to enjoy nature, exercise and go for walks. Make sure you have at least one fun event scheduled with your partner and some joyful time with a friend or two. Schedule in flextime to be used for whatever pops up in your life and to avoid over booking yourself.

Plan Your Work Life to Support Your Pregnancy

*In an easy and relaxed manner, in a healthy and
positive way, in its own perfect time.*

~ Marc Allen

The majority of women in North America work right up until they give birth. If you plan to do the same, it is important to determine if your work environment is a health risk to you or the baby.

For example, working in an environment with chemicals or poor air quality will present many risks to the developing fetus. If your job requires you to be exposed to chemicals, sit or stand for long periods of time, lift heavy objects or navigate around crowded areas, work with your employer to find solutions to ensure you are not stressing your body or the baby.

It is also important to get informed about your working rights while pregnant. Go online and research legislation in your area on pregnancy discrimination, protection, maternity and parental leave, medical leave and job security.

How to Stay Safe at Work
- Monitor your body and mind for signs of stress.
- Take frequent breaks to rest throughout the workday.
- Drink plenty of water.
- Eat healthy meals.
- Work regular hours and avoid working over time.
- Avoid sitting or standing for long periods of time.
- Avoid contact with chemicals.

- If your job requires stressful travel, make other arrangements.

- Reduce non-work commitments to ensure you are getting the rest you need.

- If you find yourself overwhelmed physically, request modified tasks or alternative assignments.

Establish a Departure Date From Work

If you don't design your own life plan, chances are you'll fall into someone else's plan. And guess what they have planned for you? Not much.

~ *Jim Rohn*

Investigate your company's policies on maternity leave, extended maternity leave, medical benefits and holiday entitlement. Also research maternity leave legislation in your state or province. Speak with other women in your workplace who have taken maternity leave to learn from their experiences. Have a discussion with your partner about how much time you can afford in addition to the paid time that will be covered by your employer. Determine if your partner will also be taking leave.

Once you've gathered all available information on maternity leave, determine when you'd like your leave to begin, taking into consideration the unpredictability of the actual due date. Then notify your employer of your pregnancy and your planned departure date for maternity leave with a written notice of intention to take maternity leave.

Begin making a list of job responsibilities that will need to be handled by someone else when you are on leave. Ensure all passwords and access to

241

accounts and information is available. If you are part of a long-term project, ensure everyone who shares the project or is influenced by the project knows you will be on leave for a portion of the project.

Ask if there are flexible work arrangements available to transition back to work around the number of days per week you'd like to work. Let your employer know when you'd like to return to work, but be realistic in determining your return date.

Take a Leave of Absence

If men got pregnant...maternity leave would last two years with full pay.

~ Unknown

If complications occur or you are feeling overwhelmed physically or mentally during your pregnancy, then follow the advice of your health practitioner and take time off work to take care of yourself. In North America, if you need to leave work early as a result of pregnancy complications or discomfort you are entitled to claim disability support.

If you are financially unable to take time off, then speak with your employer about any work related concerns that may be affecting your physical or mental health. Educate yourself about your pregnancy and parental work rights and leave benefits in your state or province.

Make Up Your Mind

When we think of failure; failure will be ours. If we remain undecided; nothing will ever change. All we need to do is want to achieve something great and then simply to do it. Never think of failure, for what we think, will come about.

~ Maharishi Mahesh Yogi

Sitting on the fence for long periods of time can be painful and stressful. Indecision often occurs because we fear and doubt our decisions and lack self-confidence. It can be debilitating and can result in missed opportunities and regret. Using indecisiveness to keep you from potential rejection or from facing a fear is a type of self-sabotage. When you come to the end of your life are you going to reflect on what you've done or regret what you haven't? Henry Ford simplified the issue when he said, "Indecision is often worse than wrong action."

The key to decision making when you feel stuck is to follow your instinct. If you need some practice, try quick decision making with the small stuff like choosing a menu item or what you are going to wear for the day. Allow your intuition to guide you. Once you've made a decision, trust it. Enjoy the experiences your choice has brought. Learn from any choices that were less than ideal. Winston Churchill once said, "Success is not final, failure is not fatal: it is the courage to continue that counts."

If you are having difficulties deciding between two options, ask yourself a few questions:

- What is the worst thing that can happen if I choose X?
- What is the worst thing that can happen if I choose Y?

243

- What is the best thing that can happen if I choose X?
- What is the best thing that can happen if I choose Y?
- Can you deal with the consequences of choosing one decision over another?

Another technique is to list your options. Brainstorm all the possible outcomes and consequences of each possibility. Determine your ultimate outcome for your decision. Which of your options most likely fits with your desired outcome?

If you are still having difficulties deciding, try bouncing your dilemma off of a friend or your partner. Talking to someone may assist you to see the situation from another perspective.

Ultimately, if waiting to decide something feels stressful, get off the fence and decide. Sometimes this takes setting aside some time for reflection and may even require you putting a time limit on the decision making process.

Sing

There's no half-singing in the shower,
you're either a rock star or an opera diva.

~ *Josh Groban*

Whether it is in the shower or in the car, singing can be a great way to make you feel better. Not only is singing a superb stress reducer, it actually has a number of physical and emotional benefits such as decreasing the effects of depression, exercises your heart and lungs, and improves your posture. In addition, singing improves circulation, releases pain relieving endorphins, energizes the body and boosts the immune system. Choose songs with positive messages and that leave you feeling uplifted. With so many benefits to singing, why not take the opportunity to sing today!

Wear Something Colorful

Color is joy. One does not think joy.

One is carried by it.

~ Ernst Haas

Color is highly influential on our moods and experiences. Brightly painted yellow doors decorate many houses in Ireland. In a country that receives more than its fair share of dreary grey days, the Irish use bright colored paint on their doors to lift their mood and to counter the effects of so much dullness.

The power of color reaches us in different ways and infuses our psychology. Certain colors become associated with your life experiences in subtle and subconscious ways. Consequently, the meaning you attribute to color and how you are affected by color is different than how others interpret and experience color.

Wearing different colors can greatly affect how you feel in any given day. It may be as simple as accessorizing with a colorful scarf or you may be inspired to wear a colorful blouse or dress. Although we all have our own sense of style, explore the more colorful side of your style while you are pregnant. Choose colors that you associate with feeling inspired and fabulous. Also, experiment with a color you have never worn before and see how it changes your mood.

Although color affects people in different ways, there are certain attributes associated with particular colors that you may like to reflect on:

- *Pink* - Unconditional Love. Flowers are the biggest natural influence of pink in our lives. The pink lotus is often associated with the color of compassion and unconditional love. Although pink was originally a color associated with baby boys (because of is relationship to red), since the 1940's it has been marketed as a girl color.

- *Red* - Stimulation. Red is associated with warmth, blood, fire, danger, passion and love. In North America, red has been used in traffic to represent the signal to stop. Over time, this has a subtle and subconscious affect on our relationship to the color red. In Chinese culture, red is associated with good luck. Red ochre is associated with the sacred and secret.

- *Orange* - Inspiring. Orange is known as a healing and powerful color that is often associated with fall. Spices, oranges, pumpkins, sunsets and Buddhist robes are just some of the influences of orange in our life.

- *Yellow* - Refreshing. The yellow hues of the sun inspire joy, aliveness and energy. If you are feeling down, yellow may be just the color you need to nourish you.

- *Green* - Stress Reliever. If we are lucky, we live in areas that are filled with green grass, plants and trees. Green is linked to reducing stress and it is believed to increase one's memory. Spending time in a natural green space is a great way to infuse peace into ones body and mind. Green also represents health and wellness.

- *Blue* - Calming. The blue colors of sky and water have beautifully influenced our minds. Often associated with cooling and calmness, the color blue is a perfect choice to encourage relaxation.

- *Purple* - Creativity. It is believed that purple brings to mind authority, wisdom, spiritual fulfillment, magic, mystery and royalty. Since purple is a combination of blue and red, it both dynamic and calming, purple cultivates creativity and inspiration.

- *Brown* - Strength. Brown shows up in the color of the earth and wood. Feelings of strength and grounding are often associated with brown, so it makes it a perfect color when need a boost of strength.

Be Creative

May your mind whirl joyful cartwheels of creativity.
May your heart sing sweet lullabies of timelessness.
May your essence be the nectar of the open blossom of your joy.
May your spirit soar throughout the vast cathedral of your being.

~ *Jonathan Lockwood Huie*

Creative activities, such as art design, art making, video or sound creation, movement and exploring the imagination, can offer an opportunity to relax, quiet the mind and inspire insight around stressful life experiences which in turn helps to relieve stress and trigger healing. On an emotional level, creativity gives us an outlet to experience our emotions in a healthy way. In addition, creativity builds confidence and has a positive effect on our self-esteem.

Creativity also offers many benefits for our brain. It has been linked to increased memory, neural stimulation and better brain function. The better our brain functions, the better we are at dealing with the different sources of stresses in our life.

If you find it challenging to be creative, I have included some ways that you can get your creative juices flowing:

- ✓ *Take some time for you.* The first step is to always take time for yourself to relax. Go for a walk, read a book, get some sleep – do something that helps you unwind. Once you feel relaxed, you will find that your creative juices are flowing and you'll have more energy to give to that creativity.

- ✓ *Design your space.* Go to baby stores, look through magazines and design books and then create a space for you or your baby's nursery.

- ✓ *Mind map the possibilities.* A mind map is a brainstorming diagram that you draw to represent your words, tasks or ideas. The map is organized in an intuitive and radial design that mirrors the neural connections in the brain. Mind maps work brilliantly to generate solutions or clarify ideas or even to structure and organize them. It is a creative, simple and fun process that uses color and images. Do an online search on "mind maps" for inspiration for making your own mind maps.

- ✓ *Be grateful for what you have.* The best moments of creativity sometimes come right after you have acknowledged all the current blessings in your life. Gratitude creates a wave of positive energy that spirals into a greater level of creativity.

✓ *Take an art class.* Find a local class and let yourself be guided into a creative activity in a setting that provides support for cultivating your creativity.

✓ *Find inspiration in the little things.* Notice, collect and store inspirational images, objects or notes you come across in your day. When you have time, pull your treasures out and allow them to inspire your creative activity.

Make Time to Bond With Your Friends

Repeated exposures to the people with whom we feel the closest social bonds can condition the release of oxytocin, so that merely being in their presence, or even just thinking about them, may trigger in us a pleasant dose.

~ *Dan Goleman, Social Intelligence*

The hormones associated with pregnancy have a tendency to encourage nesting. Regardless of the tendency to want to stick around home, it is important to continue to nurture bonding and fun activities with friends to reduce stress, keep relationships healthy and to access the many benefits of friendship.

We all know how it feels to spend fun time with girlfriends. The time with gal pals provide fun experiences, laughter, support and nurturing in ways that our partner may not be able to offer. If you need a listening ear, friends are a great sounding board and unconditional support for issues you may need to express. Schedule at least one girlfriend outing a month. If possible, plan a fun event ever week.

Buy Something for You

When women are depressed, they eat or go shopping. Men invade another country.
It's a whole different way of thinking.

~ Elayne Boosler

Everyone enjoys buying a little something for themselves from time to time. Generally, throughout pregnancy, the focus is on what needs to be purchased for the baby or the house, but we often forget to take care of ourselves. Take time from your schedule to go out and find a gift that is perfect for you. When you do go out to buy something special for yourself, make a day of it and invite a friend to enjoy the experience with you.

Shopping can help relieve stress but only if it is not at the expense of your budget and only if you are feeling joyful while doing it. Shop within your budget, but free yourself from thinking the money should be spent on someone or something else.

Buy a Specialty Pillow

I had suffered from awful back and hip pain from the beginning of my second trimester.
My husband surprised me with a body pillow and I instantly fell in love with it.

~ Anonymous

While pregnant, using a specialty pillow is a great way to help alleviate physical stress, prevent back pain and to get a restful sleep. When you choose a pillow, there are a number of different types that you could consider. I recommend as natural a pillow as possible. Avoid pillows that have been infused with antimicrobial chemicals, as they can be harmful to you and the baby. The level of comfort that you get from each type of pillow will differ depending on your own preference.

- *Knee Pillows* - Designed to fit between your knees when you lay on your side, a knee pillow helps align the spine and supports the pelvis. This type of pillow can help prevent back pain and will also help correct misalignment in your hips.

- *Neck Pillows* - Engineered to fill the space under the head and neck, a neck pillow or cervical pillow helps create proper alignment of your neck with your spine and can offer that extra support needed for a good night's rest.

- *Body Pillows* - Designed to follow the natural contours of your whole body, a full body pillow can offer relief from physical pain associated with pregnancy while sleeping at night. The body pillow offers support for the back and helps to minimize back pain. The added bonus for pregnant women is that the pillow can be placed under the belly to provide abdominal support as they lay on their side.

- *Under the Knee Pillow* - If you are at the beginning stage of pregnancy and can still lie on your back when you sleep, I highly recommend placing a small pillow under your knees for additional comfort and to alleviate strain on the lower back.

The hardness of the pillow can differ and it really depends on your personal preference but a good guideline is to give a pillow about a week. If, after a week, you still don't find it comfortable, return it and purchase a new pillow until you find the perfect one that makes you feel at ease.

Get Your Daily Hugs

We need four hugs a day for survival. We need eight hugs a day for maintenance.
We need twelve hugs a day for growth.

~ Virgina Satir

Touch is an essential need for the body and mind. We thrive on physical touch and without it people often suffer from physical and mental health problems. Children are natural at hugging and cuddling, but as adults, we often get busy with day-to-day activities and forget about connecting through touch.

I recommend that you make time for at least five hugs per day. Oxytocin is released after about 20 seconds, so linger longer when you hug your partner, family or friends. Shorter hugs don't have the same effect. If you haven't hugged anyone lately, create an opportunity to get those hugs in now! Here are some benefits to getting hugged today:

- **Reduction of cortisol.** Research shows that hugging lowers cortisol (a stress hormone) and reduces stress on the body.

- **Reduced risk of heart disease and stroke.** Hugging does the heart good and it can also help prevent heart disease by lowering blood pressure.

- **Improved intimacy.** Hugging your partner, family member or a friend provides an opportunity for each person to know that they are loved.

- **Reduced anxiety.** When another embraces us it allows us to feel safe, more secure, not so alone and less anxious.

- **Helps us relax.** Hugging helps us relax by releasing a cascade of feel good chemicals such as oxytocin.

Journal

Sometime in your life you will go on a journey.
It will be the longest journey you have ever taken.
It is the journey to find yourself.

~ *Katherine Sharp*

Journaling is all about keeping a written account of your thoughts and feelings surrounding the events of your life, your dreams and your pregnancy. It is an inexpensive and meaningful tool for self-exploration and transformation.

One of the biggest benefits of journaling is that subconscious beliefs or unconscious emotions have a vehicle for expression. When more information is revealed, it empowers you through self-knowledge to heal, to bring awareness to a situation that you may not have been fully conscious of, or to clarify your thoughts and emotions.

Also, journaling helps you to process trauma, to put issues into perspective, to reduce stress and it provides an outlet for expressing challenging emotions such as anger and sadness.

Health Benefits

Researchers have found that students who write about their emotions and thoughts, related to a trauma or stress, develop a greater awareness of the positive benefits of the stressful event. Those who wrote only about their negative emotions without writing their reflections tended to report more illness than other participants.[208] However, for people who have severe anxiety disorders, journaling has been shown to be less successful unless it is paired with the guidance and care of a health care provider.

Studies have also revealed that expressive writing has a beneficial effect on people's physical and mental health including less visits to the doctor, reduced stress, alleviation of depression, an increased positive outlook, improved immune functioning, lower heart rates and blood pressure, faster healing after surgery, a decrease of asthma and arthritis symptoms and a reduction in stress-related physical symptoms.

How to Journal

I love writing with a pen and paper, but everyone has their preferences. You can journal in a cheap notebook, an ornate journal or on a computer. Interestingly, one study revealed that hand writing emotional narratives about a stressful experience tends to illicit more disclosure compared to typing.

Journal whenever you feel drawn to write or set aside a specific time at the end of the day. I like to journal when I first wake up in the morning and I often incorporate a dream that I have had before waking up.

When journaling dreams, I first write the full account of the dream as though it is happening as I write. I include my feelings and emotional states. Once I have finished writing the dream, I take a short break from it and return to it later. I am often surprised to learn a great deal from my dream that I didn't see before and I make note of the wisdom I've learned.

I also use journaling to write down favorite quotes or inspirations from my day. Sometimes I draw pictures or glue photographs or images from magazines into my journal.

When you sit down to journal, write continuously for at least fifteen minutes. If you think that is too long, commit to at least five minutes and do it. You'd be surprised at how fast five minutes goes by.

You can write about anything that comes to mind. Similarly, you can do one exercise that goes like this: Write every thought that comes into your mind about any issue or stress affecting your life. Continue to write until there is nothing left to write about the situation.

Other Journaling Suggestions:

- Write about your stresses, how you feel about them and even what you think the solutions may be.
- Write for you and nobody else.
- If it helps play some relaxing and healing music, but choose music without lyrics as the words can easily influence your subconscious mind.
- Include journaling about gratitude. A simple exercise is to list five experiences, people or things you are grateful for each day.
- If you have a secret you want to write about, try journaling imaginary words about it with your finger. One study reported that similar beneficial results are achieved when you write with a pen on paper or if you pretend to write with your finger.

Spend Time Watching the Stars & Moon

Learn to get in touch with the silence within yourself and
know that everything in life has a purpose.

~ Elisabeth Kubler-Ross

Spending time gazing at the stars or a full moon is a wonderful way to enjoy an evening. Whether it is a romantic time with your partner, a fun time with friends or a solitary experience of contemplating the universe, relax and allow the light of the celestial bodies to calm your mind. When you simply look up at the night sky, inhale a cleansing breath and then release it dispelling whatever stress you are willing to give over to the universe. If it has been a while since you gazed at the heavens, grab a warm blanket and get outside to enjoy the magic.

Drink a Cup of Herbal Tea & Daydream

Each cup of tea represents an imaginary voyage.

~ Catherine Douzel

A simple but powerful strategy for having a stress free pregnancy is to simply create quiet moments to sit down, relax and enjoy a soothing cup of herbal tea. Take time to sit with yourself and enjoy the peaceful moment. Gaze out a window and watch nature. If it is nice enough outside, take your tea and sit in the fresh air. Daydream. Have a conversation with your baby. Allow for the ease of the moment to entrain you into relaxation. Breathe.

Herbal teas can be enjoyed hot on cool days. However, you can cool brewed tea the in the refrigerator and serve it cold on warm sunny days. I suggest avoiding using ice as it waters down the flavor of the tea, kills beneficial bacteria in your digestive system and drains energy from the body.

Caffeine crosses the placenta and reaches your developing baby who cannot metabolize caffeine like an adult. Herbal teas are naturally caffeine free, so explore the herbal options and find some new favorites. Avoid caffeinated teas such as black, green or white tea.

Drinking certain herbal teas is a great way to support your prenatal health as many herbal teas provide nutrients and minerals, however not all herbal teas are safe during your pregnancy. All herbal teas must be consumed in moderation. Talk with your midwife, nutritionist, herbalist or doctor about more helpful herbal teas to drink during pregnancy.

Supportive Teas

Some of the safest herbal teas that calm the nervous system include

- **Ginger** – Ginger helps to relieve nausea and vomiting. It also stimulates digestion. Since ginger tends to be stimulating, avoid drinking it in the evenings.
- **Lemon balm** – This herb has a calming effect that helps relieve irritability, insomnia and anxiety.
- **Nettle leaf** – A great source of iron, vitamins and minerals. Drink no more than a cup per day. Avoid excess consumption in the first trimester.
- **Peppermint leaf** – Aids digestion and helps to relieve nausea and flatulence.
- **Pregnancy tea** – Various herbal tea companies have created

pregnancy teas. Teas can be purchased online or in organic groceries.

- **Red raspberry leaf** – This herbal tea is the safest of all uterine and pregnancy herbs. High in iron, vitamins and minerals, red raspberry leaf tea tonifies the pelvic muscles and the uterus, eases morning sickness, reduces birth pain, reduces incidences of forceps delivery and cesarean birth and assists in the production of breast milk. In addition, red raspberry leaf has been used to treat an upset stomach, acne, diarrhea, vomiting, menstrual issues, inflammation and gum disease. In the first trimester, doctors recommend you limit yourself to one cup per day.

- **Roasted barley** – Also known as Mugicha, this herbal tea is high in antioxidants. It is also an antibacterial, assists in breaking up congestion and phlegm, is good for blood circulation and helps reduce blood toxicity.

- **Rose hips** – High in Vitamin C.

- **Rooibos** – High in antioxidants, rooibos has been known to relieve aches and pains during pregnancy, is an anti-inflammatory, aids in digestion, helps heal skin conditions, prevents cancer, helps control blood sugar levels and much more.

Teas to Avoid (partial list)

- Black, green, white, orange pekoe, Earl Grey and oolong – These teas have caffeine and are associated with blocking folic acid uptake, which has detrimental effects on fetal health.

- Burdock root, chamomile, chicory, comfrey, ephedra, fennel, hibiscus, horehound, Labrador, licorice root, mistletoe, mugwart, pennyroyal, rosemary, sage, sassafras, large amounts of stinging nettle, vetiver, yarrow, yellow dock and yerba mate.

258

Meditate to Calm the Mind & Body

The soul loves to meditate, for in contact with the Spirit lies its greatest joy. If, then you experience mental resistance during meditation, remember that reluctance to meditate comes from the ego; it doesn't belong to the soul.

~ *Paramahansa Yogananda*

Meditation is a great strategy for reducing stress, cultivating relaxation, slowing cellular aging, improving memory, decreasing anxiety, alleviating depression and calming the mind. Even 15 minutes a day can have a significant effect on your health. One study found that mindfulness based stress reduction, using meditation and gentle yoga, assisted pregnant women to reduce perceived stress and depression, as well as improve well-being.[209]

Meditation has also been found to lower blood pressure, lower the risk of pre-eclampsia, reduce cesarean surgeries, prevent preterm birth and reduce stress hormones that might be detrimental to the fetus. Thomas Verny, author of *Tomorrow's Baby* shares that "...maternal feelings and moods are linked to hormones and neurotransmitters that travel through the bloodstream and across the placenta to the developing brain of the unborn child."[210] The biological and physiological benefits of meditation are transmitted to the fetus via hormones and neurotransmitters. If you haven't tried meditation, look for a class in your area.

Use Creative Visualization to Calm
the Mind & Body

Visualization is daydreaming with a purpose.

~ Bo Bennett

Creative visualization is an effective way to relax the mind and body and induce a peaceful state. Since the mind cannot tell the difference between an actual event and an imagined one, visualization can be like a mini-holiday. Using a stress relieving strategy, such as creative visualization, can lower blood pressure and reduce stress hormones. It is also a great way to get in touch with your intuition and to cultivate creativity.

You can use your own imagination or listen to a downloaded guided meditation. When using your imagination, visualize yourself at a beach, in a meadow or in an imaginary space that has all the elements of safety, love, peace, aliveness and nourishment that you can imagine. You can swim with dolphins, fly through the air or just lounge in the sunshine by a waterfall. You can even meet and interact with your baby. You may want to listen to relaxing music at the same time or just allow your imagination to create whatever sound you'd like to hear. I prefer to lie down when I do creative visualizations, but you can do them sitting up or in whatever position is comfortable to you.

Learn Guided Relaxation Techniques

When you change the way you view birth, the way you birth will change.

~ Marie F. Mongan

Maternal stress and negative moods, such as anxiety and depression, increase risk to developing fetuses. Guided relaxation exercises are easy to learn and are effective ways to reduce stress and anxiety. Guided relaxation is the practice of listening to a recording of a human voice, often combined with music, to guide you into a relaxed state. This is a similar process to guided meditation. In research on stress management during pregnancy, expecting women have reported many benefits to guided relaxation.[211] Some of those benefits include:

- Improved breathing
- The ability to experience calm, relaxation and mental clarity
- Reduction of stress and anxiety
- Reduction of anger
- Increased ability to fall asleep and to sleep through the night

You can purchase guided relaxation CDs in stores or download them online. There are many to choose from. However, the most popular among expecting women are the Hypnobabies or Hypnobirthing classes, books and CDs. Hypnobabies and Hypnobirthing are effective relaxation techniques that use self-hypnosis or self-guided relaxation combined with natural birthing education for the purpose of experiencing a safer, more peaceful, energized birthing experience with fewer complications and chemical painkillers.

The major difference between Hypnobabies and Hypnobirthing is that Hypnobabies uses medical hypno-anesthesia techniques to support the mom to have a pain free birthing experience with eyes open, moving around or talking. Whereas Hypnobirthing teaches relaxation techniques for a more comfortable birthing while staying still with eyes closed. There are courses and trained practitioners available throughout North America and around the world.

Develop Mindfulness

Mindfulness means paying attention in a particular way;
on purpose, in the present moment, and nonjudgmentally.

~ Jon Kabat-Zinn

Mindfulness is a practice of awareness for the benefit of improving your clarity and equanimity. In the beginning you may practice awareness for a short time each day, but the goal or intention is to carry mindfulness into everything you do. Eventually, the embodied state of clarity and equanimity become deeply ingrained into your consciousness and every aspect of your life.

The benefit of practicing mindfulness is that it can assist you to be free from the suffering of emotional, physical and spiritual discomfort even when challenges arise. It also assists people to feel fulfilled and peaceful regardless of the circumstances they find themselves in. In addition, mindfulness is a powerful way to increase your ability to concentrate and focus on what is important in the moment. In recent research, mindfulness based practices have significantly shown a decrease in anxiety and negative mood.[212]

How to Practice Mindfulness

There are two types of mindfulness practices you may want to try:

- **Simple Sitting Mediation** - Start a sitting meditation practice where you sit upright with your eyes open or closed for 20 minutes each day. Sit cross-legged with your hips above your knees for comfort or sit in a chair with your knees at a 90-degree angle and your feet on the ground. Allow your hands to rest together on your lap. If your eyes are open, let your gaze fall unfocused upon the floor or ground a few feet in front of you. Let your gaze be relaxed and soft. Always keep your tongue on the roof of your mouth to connect the flow of energy through your main energy meridian. Breathe in and out through your nose. With soft focus, be mindful of your breath as it flows in and out of your body. If thoughts arise, bring your attention back to the breath.

- **Everyday Mindfulness** - Practice bringing mindfulness to every moment of your day. When you wake up in the morning, bring awareness to your body and how you move into the world. While brushing your teeth, washing your face or having a shower, be present for each experience in that moment. Connect fully with your partner when you encounter each other. If ever you feel overwhelmed in any circumstance, bring your attention to your breath and heart centre. Be mindful in all situations, whether it is doing the dishes, taking a walk, pumping gas or eating a meal. If thoughts arise that are not related to the activity you are doing, just let them go.

Slow down as you move through your day and enjoy every moment of your pregnancy. Remember to make space for mindfulness throughout your day by taking breaks, listening to the sounds around you and enjoying the colors and textures you see. Observe all aspects of your life. Let go of expectations. See the world as it is, without any story from you.

If you are having a particularly busy day, take calming breaths, close your eyes and allow yourself moments of calm every hour. Even five minutes of calm will refresh you and will get you back into the tasks at hand. You and your baby will benefit greatly.

Open Your Heart

Love is the light that dissolves all walls between souls, families and nations.

~ *Paramahansa Yogananda*

Our spiritual heart is our center of love and compassion. In many spiritual traditions, the heart center (or heart chakra) is the seat of the soul.

Why Open Your Heart?

Opening your heart is a path to experiencing a life of peace, joy, compassion and aliveness. By learning to listen to your heart you access and connect with your soul wisdom, which assists you to make decisions for your highest good and greatest joy.

Why Does the Heart Close?

The heart often closes when negative feelings become repressed and emotions become too overwhelming to deal with. A closed heart most likely stems from past trauma, often from early childhood, but can happen at any point in a person's life.

The primary reason that emotions become too difficult to face is because they arise from a belief or series of beliefs that are created by the ego mind, which is the root cause of most of our suffering and delusions. The ego mind begins developing around the age of three years when children start learning codes of behavior, defenses and ways to survive and function effectively according to the environment into which the child is born.

Although it is hoped that a healthy ego will develop, many children grow into adults with fears of rejection, abandonment, shame, guilt and inferiority. From experiences of pain and suffering, the ego develops strategies to protect one from shame or pain. However, the strategies are maladapted and tend to create the very situation the ego tries to convince you to avoid. The attempt to keep the pain out also keeps the pain in.

When you believe the false thoughts the ego tells you, that you are under attack and have to defend yourself, you set yourself up for suffering. Ultimately the ego convinces you to give up your power to the idea that you are weak. This is a type of influence you allow from your own mind.

Realize that other people's behavior is not a personal attack against you; it is a personal attack against them. What they say about you, or how they treat you, is an indication of what is in their heart. Choose to be free of the influence of what others believe about themselves or you. When you believe what they say or do as a personal reflection of you, you close your heart to you. You are causing your own pain. You have chosen to allow their influence, to believe their fantasy and to close your heart to yourself. Instead,

265

have compassion for the pain they must be feeling to express themselves in such a negative way.

You can still reflect on what they have said. Maybe there is some wisdom about you in their expression of pain and suffering. If so, reflect mindfully without judgment toward yourself and use what you learn to live your life with an open heart, to heal your life and bring light into the world.

How to Open the Heart

There are many techniques for opening the heart. I'll share a simple method below. But first, set the intention for you to make a heart centered commitment to living the deepest truth of who you are, even if you don't yet know who you are. Trust in the beauty and wisdom of you unfolding in your lifetime.

Exercise for Opening the Heart:

- With your eyes open, see the room as it is. Become present in the moment. See everything as it is, free from the judgments and ideas of your mind. With the beginning of acceptance of what is, you can begin to accept you as you are.
- Take a deep breath in through your nose expanding your belly. Exhale through your mouth and make a 'Haaaaaah' noise. Do this three times. Then breathe normally, gently inhaling and exhaling through the nose.
- Bring your attention to your heart center.
- Smile to your heart center.
- Gently place your hand over the heart center.
- Keep smiling to your heart.

- Connect with the source of Love within by asking the wisdom and intelligence of your heart center to assist you to open your heart to Love, to heal any pain or negative emotions, and to guide you to express and receive love more fully.
- Visualize Divine Light flowing from above you, in through the top of your head and filling your heart center.
- Ask the Divine Light to bless and purify your heart of all negative beliefs, attitudes and emotions, so that you can open your heart to yourself and others.
- Ask the Divine Light to forgive you for any pain or suffering that you have created for yourself and others.
- Ask the Divine Light to forgive anyone for any pain or suffering that they have caused you.
- Say thank you to the wisdom and intelligence of your heart center and to the Divine Light.
- Continue smiling to your heart center.
- Everyday, bring love to every situation by surrendering everything to the heart center: all your ideas, emotions and impressions.
- Choose to be vulnerable, real and true to yourself.
- Choose to embody love regardless of the situation you find yourself in.

I offer you peace. I offer you love. I offer you friendship.
I see your beauty. I hear your need. I feel your feelings.
My wisdom flows from the Highest Source. I salute that Source in you.
Let us work together for unity and love.
~ Gandhi

Conclusion

I 've shared over 100 ways you can cultivate peace in your pregnancy. When dealing with stress of any kind, it is not always easy to navigate through the emotions and side effects associated with stress. The key to achieving less stress is to apply the strategies that work best for you and to be consistent with applying them. Be adventurous; try some of the techniques I have suggested, especially Emotional Freedom Technique.

EFT is one of those tools that you can apply in every area of your life, for the rest of your life. It is also a great tool to teach your children, to assist them with anything that triggers stress as they grow and learn. My hope for you is that you will feel empowered by the changes you can implement to reduce or eliminate stress by using the suggested strategies in this book. Then use these strategies beyond your pregnancy to create a stress free life.

There are many women who rely on others to lead them on their prenatal journey. This is your journey! You are entrusted to be more conscious about designing how your pregnancy unfolds. Enjoying a peaceful, stress free pregnancy necessitates courage, choice, responsibility, growth and patience. Celebrate this responsibility! You have the power to make powerful and positive changes to your life that will nourish both you and your baby.

If you'd like further inspiration or encouragement on cultivating a peaceful pregnancy, contact me or sign up for a session or one of my courses. I am available to serve you in whatever way I can.

We need to teach the next generation of children from day one that they are responsible for their lives. Mankind's greatest gift, also its greatest curse, is that we have free choice. We can make our choices built from love or from fear.

~ Elisabeth Kubler-Ross

Recommended Resources

Positive Birthing Videos

- Orgasmic Birth DVD directed by Debra Pascali-Bonaro (2008)
- The Business of Being Born DVD directed by Abby Epstein (2008)
- Birth As We Know It DVD directed by Elena Tonetti-Vladimirova (2006)
- Birth Day DVD directed by Diana Paul and Frank Ferrel (2008)
- The Face of Birth DVD directed by Kate Gorman and Gavin Banks (2012)
- Youtube videos with keywords 'hypnobabies water birth'

Pregnancy and Childbirth Books

- Pregnancy, Childbirth, and the Newborn by Simkin, Walley, Keppler, Durham & Bolding (2010)
- Sacred Birthing: Birthing a New Humanity by Sunni Karll (2003)
- Orgasmic Birth by Elizabeth Davis & Debra Pascali-Bonaro (2010)
- Ina May's Guide to Childbirth by Ina May Gaskin (2010)
- Childbirth Without Fear by Grantly Dick-Read, Foreword by Ina May Gaskin (2013)

Childbirth Education

- Stress Free Pregnancy - www.stress-free-pregnancy.com
- Hypnobabies - www.hypnobabies.com
- Hypnobirthing - www.hypnobirthing.com
- Birthing from Within - www.birthingfromwithin.com
- Lamaze International – www.lamaze.org
- The Bradley Method - www.bradleybirth.com/

To Find a Doula or a Midwife

- DONA International - www.dona.org
- CAPPA - www.cappa.net
- Childbirth International - www.childbirthinternational.com
- To find a midwife in your area, do a search online for local midwife associations.

Breastfeeding Books & Support

- Womanly Art of Breastfeeding by La Leche League International (2010)
- Breastfeeding Answers Made Simple: Seven Natural Laws for Nursing Mothers by Nancy Mohrbacher (2010)
- La Leche League International - www.llli.org/

Newborn Parenting Resources

- Attached at the Heart by Barbara Nicholson and Lysa Parker (2009)
- The Attachment Connection by Ruth P Newton (2008)
- The No Cry Sleep Solution by Elizabeth Pantly (2002)
- The Baby Book: Everything You Need to Know About Your Baby from Birth to Age Two by William Sears and Martha Sears (2003)
- The Continuum Concept by Jean Liedloff (1977)
- Magical Child by Joseph Chilton Pearce (1992)
- Attachment Parenting International - www.attachmentparenting.org

Acknowledgements

With deep gratitude I thank everyone who has ever touched my life. Weaving in and around and through it all, the Divine has gifted me the unfolding of such a beautiful and interesting life. Thank you, dearest Divine, for inspiring me to see the importance of a peaceful pregnancy, birthing and parenting for the birthing of a new humanity.

I am grateful for all my teachers, throughout my existence for your support and love. To Master Dhyan Vimal for your guidance to be free of influence. To Master Peter Huboba for embodying the pure love of the Divine Mother. To Lynn Mundel for teaching me the simple and powerful blessing of presence.

To the pioneers and advocates of childbirth education who have touched the hearts of birthing women and have inspired peaceful births. Some of these wonderful people include Dr. Grantly Dick-Read, Penny Simkin, Ina May Gaskin, Dr Michel Odent, Dr. Marshall H. Klaus, John Kennell, Pam England, Kathie Lindstrom, Sunni Karll and many more celebrated and anonymous men and women. To Dr. Bruce Lipton for your inspirational work in epigenetics.

To my amazing family who helped shape who I am. Thank you Kelly for your encouragement and love, for believing in me in ways that deeply touch my heart. To Jenny for your deep compassion for others and animals. To my Dad who sees my potential and taught me stick-to-it-ness and to take care of what needs to be done. To my Mom for birthing me and having the wisdom to ask God to look after and guide me throughout my life. A beautiful gift!

To John for your loving, open-hearted support and patience on my ever-evolving adventure into life. Thank you for believing in me.

To Mark for your unwavering devotion, nourishment and assistance in supporting me in completing this book.

To Bobby and Rachel for your contributions to the book.

To you, the reader of this book, for making a difference in the world by cultivating peace within you and for your child to be.

About the Author

*T*ara Bianca is a spiritual and transformational coach, facilitator and author whose inspirational mentorship empowers everyday people to transform their lives to access joy, aliveness, clarity, focus and direction.

Her passion is inspired by her own transformation when, after many years of incredible emotional and spiritual suffering, her physical health unraveled. Recognizing the power of responsibility and presence, she discovered a pathway to peace and joy. Since then she has dedicated her life to assisting those who are ready to live an intentional and extraordinary life of joy.

Her book *Stress Free Pregnancy* is an important step in assisting parents to birth babies freer of stress than previous generations, so that these children have the opportunity to excel in life. The book was inspired by two discoveries. The first discovery was that most of her clients' core issues stemmed from their parents' stress and suffering. The second revelation was the rising number of pregnant women who suffered from stress, depression and anxiety.

After obtaining a B.A. Degree, Tara had a business background in operational management before spending seven years as a nutritional researcher, coach and personal living foods chef to celebrities. She also served as a cofounder and board member of the Raw Food Society of BC.

Currently, Tara is a writer, speaker, coach and consultant for transformational aliveness. Her multidisciplinary approaches and methods guide people through quantum shifts to access their ability to create a life from an entirely different level of consciousness and to be a source of inspiration for others in the world. She writes about transformation, aliveness, consciousness, pregnancy and nutrition.

Connect with Tara: **www.tarabianca.com**

www.stress-free-pregnancy.com

Citations

1 O'Hare T, Creed F. Life events and miscarriage. *Br J Psychiatry* (1995) Dec; 167 (6): 799-805.

2 Maconochie N, Doyle P, Prior S, Simmons R. Risk factor for first trimester miscarriage-results from a UK-population-based case control study. *BJOG* (2007) Feb; 114(2): 170-186.

3 Glynn LM, Schetter CD, Hobel CJ, Sandman CA. Pattern of perceived stress and anxiety in pregnancy predicts preterm birth. *Health Psychol* (2008) Jan; 27(1): 43-51.

4 Rumbold A, Duley L, Crowther C, Haslam R. Antioxidants for preventing pre-eclampsia. *Cochrane Database Syst Rev* (2005) Oct 19; (4): CD004227.

5 Guibert F, Lumineau S, Kotrschal K, et al. Trans-generational effects of prenatal stress in quail. *Proceedings of the Royal Society of Biological Sciences* (2012) Dec; doi: 10.1098/rspb.2012.2368.

6 Kinney DK, Munir KM, Crowley DJ, Miller AM. Prenatal stress and risk for autism. *Neurosci Biobehav Rev* (2008) Oct; 32(8): 1519-1532.

7 Thomas JD, Abou EJ, Dominguez HD. Prenatal choline supplementation mitigates the adverse effects of prenatal alcohol exposure on development in rats. *Neurotoxicol Teratol* (2009) Sept-Oct; 31(5): 303-11.

8 Sharp H, Pickles A, Meaney M, Marshall K, Tibu F, et al. Frequency of infant stroking reported by mothers moderates the effect of prenatal depression on infant behavioural and physiological outcomes. *PLoS ONE* (2012) 7(10): e45446. doi: 10.1371/journal.pone.0045446.

9 Gordon I, Bennett RH, vander Wyk BC, et al. Oxytocin's impact on social cognitive brain function in youth with ASD. Oral presentation of research. International Society for Autism Research, May 19, 2012. <www.imfar.confex.com/imfar/2012/webprogram/Paper10197.html> (Accessed 13 Mar 2013).

10 Ritter-Box CM. "Breastfeeding saved my daughter's life." *Blogging for Boobs*. Sept 14, 2012. <http://www.thebreastintentions.com/1/post/2012/09/ breastfeeding-saved-my-daughters-life.html> (Accessed 5 Jan 2013).

11 *Sri Guru Granth Sahib*, M 4, p 1325.

[12] *Sri Guru Granth Sahib*, M 1, p 1030.

[13] Benor DJ, Ledger K, Toussaint L, Hett G, Zaccaro D. Pilot study of emotional freedom techniques, wholistic hybrid derived from eye movement desensitization and reprocessing and emotional freedom technique, and cognitive behavioral therapy for treatment of test anxiety in university students. *Explore (NY)*. (2009) Nov-Dec; 5(6): 338-40.

[14] Church D. The Treatment of Combat Trauma in Veterans Using EFT (Emotional Freedom Techniques): A Pilot Protocol. *Traumatology* (2010) Mar 16(1): 55-65.

[15] Napadow V, Kettner N, Hui KKS, et al. Hypothalamus and amygdala response to acupuncture stimuli in Carpal Tunnel Syndrome. *Pain* (2007) 130(3); 254-266.

[16] Akimoto T, Nakahori C, Aizawa K, Kimura F, et al. Acupuncture and responses of immunologic and endocrine markers during competition. *Medical Science and Sports Exercise* (2003); 35(8): 1296-1302.

[17] Lee S, Yin SJ, Lee ML, Tsai WJ, Sim CB. Effects of acupuncture on serum cortisol level and dopamine beta-hydroxylase activity in normal Chinese. *American Journal of Chinese Medicine* (1982); 10(1-4): 62-69.

[18] Dhond RP, Kettner N, Napadow V. Neuroimaging acupuncture effects in the human brain. *Journal of Alternative and Complementary Medicine* (2007); 13: 603-616.

[19] Fang J, Jin Z, Wang Y, et al. The salient characteristics of the central effects of acupuncture needling: limbic-paralimbic-neocortical network modulation. *Human Brain Mapping* (2009) Apr; 30(4): 1196-1206.

[20] Glazier RH, Elgar FJ, Goel V, Holzpfel S. Stress, social support, and emotional distress in a community sample of pregnant women. *J Psychosom Obstet Gynaecol* (2004) Sep-Dec; 25 (3-4): 247-55.

[21] Klaus MH, Kennell JH. The doula: an essential ingredient of childbirth rediscovered. *Acta Paediatr* (1997) Oct; 86(10): 1034-6.

[22] Nommsen-Rivers LA, Mastergeorge AM, Hansen RL, Cullum AS, Dewey KG. Doula care, early breast feeing outcomes, and breastfeeding status at 6 weeks postpartum among low-income primiparae. *J Obstet Gynecol Neonatal Nurs* (2009) Mar-Apr; 38(2): 157-73.

[23] Scott KD, Klaus PH, Klaus MH. The obstetrical and postpartum benefits of continuous support during childbirth. *Journal Womens Health Gend Based Med* (1999) Dec; 8(10): 1257-64.

[24] "What is a doula?" *Dona.org*. DONA International, n.d.
<http://www.dona.org/mothers/index.php> (Accessed 11 Nov 2011).

[25] Bellieni CV, Ceccarelli D, Rossi F, et al. Is prenatal bonding enhanced by prenatal education courses? *Minerva Gineocol* (2007) Apr; 59(2): 125-9.

[26] Lederbogen F, Kirsch P, Haddad L, et al. City living and urban upbringing affect neural social stress processing in humans. *Nature* (2011) Jun 22; 474 (7352): 498-501.

[27] Gupta JK, Hofmeyr GJ, Shehmar M. Position for women during second stage of labour for women without epidural anaesthesia. *Cochrane Database Syst Rev.* (2012) May 16; 5: CD002006.

[28] Lawrence A, Lewis L, Hofmeyr G J, Dowswell T, Styles C. Maternal positions and mobility during first stage labour. *Cochrane Database Syst Rev* (2009) Apr 15; (2): CD003934.

[29] Chen SZ, Aisaka K, Mori H, Kigawa T. Effects of sitting position on uterine activity during labor. *Obstetric Gynecology* (1987) Jan; 69(1): 67-73.

[30] McKay S. Squatting: an alternate position for the second stage of labour. *Am J Maternal Child Nur* (1984) May-June 9(3): 181-3.

[31] Gardosi J, Hutson N, B-Lynch C. Randomised, controlled trial of squatting in the second stage of labour. *Lancet* (1989) Jul 8; 2 (8654): 74-7.

[32] Bhardwaj N, Kukade J A, Patil S, & Bhardwaj S., Randomised controlled trial on modified squatting position of delivery. *Indian Journal of Maternal and Child Health* (1995) 6(2): 33-39.

[33] Gupta JK, Nikodem VC. Woman's position during second stage of labour. *Cochrane Database Syst Rev* (2000); (2): CD002006.

[34] Lieberman E, Lang JM, Frigoletto F Jr, Richardson DK, Ringer SA, Cohen A, Epidural analgesia, intrapartum fever, and neonatal sepsis evaluation. *Pediatrics* (1997); 99(3): 415-9.

[35] Anim-Somuah M, Smyth R, Howell C. Epidural versus non-epidural or no analgesia in labour. *Cochrane Database Syst Rev* (2005) Oct 19; (4): CD000331.

[36] Murray AD, Dolby RM, Nation RL, Thomas DB. Effects of epidural anesthesia on newborns and their mothers. *Child Dev* (1981); 52(1): 71-82.

[37] Zhang J, Yancey MK, Klebanoff MA et al. Does epidural analgesia prolong labor and increase risk of cesarean delivery? A natural experiment. *Am J Obstet Gynecol* (2001) Jul; 185(1): 128-34.

[38] Eberle RL, Norris MC. Labour analgesia: A risk-benefit analysis. *Drug-Saf* (1996) Apr 14(4): 239-51.

[39] Lieberman E, O'Donoghue C. Unintended effects of epidural analgesia during labor: a systematic review. *Am J Obstet Gynecol.* (2002) 186(Suppl 5): S31–68.

[40] Riordan J, Gross A, Angeron J et al. The effect of labor pain relief on neonatal suckling and breastfeeding. *J Hum Lact* (2000) Feb; 16(1): 7-12.

[41] Bodner-Adler B, Bodner K, Kimberger O, et al. The effect of epidural analgesia on the occurrence of obstetric lacerations and on the neonatal outcome during spontaneous vaginal delivery. *Arch Gynecol Obstet* (2002) Dec; 267(2): 81-4.

[42] Alstadhaug KB, Odeh F, Baloch FK, Berg DH, Salvesen R. Post-lumbar puncture headache. *Tidsskr Nor Laegeforen* (2012) Apr 17; 132(7): 818-21.

[43] Studd JW; Crawford JS; Duignan NM; Rowbotham CJ; Hughes AO. The effect of lumbar epidural analgesia on the rate of cervical dilatation and the outcome of labour of spontaneous onset. *Br J Obstet Gynaecol* (1980) 87(11): 1015-21.

[44] Anim-Somuah M, Smyth RM, Jones L. Epidural versus non-epidural or no analgesia in labour. *Cochrane Datatbase Syst Rev* (2011) Dec 7; (12): CD000331.

[45] Lieberman E, Lang J, Rigoletto F, et al. Epidural analgesia, intrapartum fever, and neonatal sepsis evaluation. *Pediatrics* (1997) Mar 1; 99(3): 415-9.

[46] Segal S. Labor epidural analgesia and maternal fever. *Anesth Analg* (2010) Dec; 111(6): 1467-75.

[47] Thorp JA, Breedlove G. Epidural analgesia in labor: an evaluation of risks and benefits. *Birth* (1996) Jun; 23(2): 63-83.

[48] Nielsen PE, Erickson JR, Abouleish EI, Perriatt S, Sheppard C. Fetal heart rate changes after intrathecal sufentanil or epidural bupivacaine for labor analgesia: incidence and clinical significance. *Anesth Analg* (1996) Oct; 83(4): 742-6.

[49] Declercq E, Menacker F, MacDorman M. Maternal risk profiles and the primary cesarean rate in the United States, 1991-2002. *Am J Public Health* (2006)b; 96: 867-72.

[50] OECD (2011), "Caesarean sections," in OECD, *Health at a Glance 2011: OECD Indicators*, OECD Publishing. doi: 10.1787/health_glance-2011-37-en.

[51] Delaney C, Cornfield DN. Risk factors for persistent pulmonary hypertension of the newborn. *Pulm Circ* (2012) Jan; 2(1): 15-20.

[52] Hyde MJ, Mostyn A, Modi N, Kemp PR. The health implications of birth by Caesarean section. *Biological Reviews* (2011) Feb; 87(1): 229-43.

[53] MacDorman MF, Declercq E, Menacker F, Malloy MH. Neonatal mortality for primary cesarean and vaginal births to low-risk women: application of an "intention-to-treat" model. *Birth* (2008) Mar; 35(1): 3-8.

[54] Azad MB, Konya T, Maughan H, et al. Gut microbiota of healthy Canadian infants: profiles by mode of delivery and infant diet at 4 months. *CMAJ* (2013) Mar 19; 185(5) 385-394.

[55] Kealy MA, Small RE, Liamputtong P. Recovery after caesarean birth: a qualitative study of women's accounts in Victoria, Australia. *BMC Pregnancy and Childbirth* (2010) 10: 47.

[56] Fitzpatrick KE, Kurinczuk JJ, Alfirevic Z, Spark P, Brocklehurst P, et al. Uterine rupture by intended mode of delivery in the UK: a national case-control study. *PLoS Med* (2012) 9(3): e1001184.

[57] Jones L, Othman M, Dowswell T, et al. Pain management for women in labour: an overview of systematic reviews. *Cochrane Database Syst Rev* (2012) Mar 14; 3: CD009234.

[58] Smith CA, Levett KM, Collins CT, Crowther CA. Relaxation techniques for pain management in labour. *Cochrane Database Syst Rev* (2011) Dec 7; (12): CD009514.

[59] Lawrence A, Lewis L, Hofmeyr GJ, Dowswell T, Styles C. Maternal positions and mobility during first stage labour. *Cochrane Databas Syst Rev* (2009) Apr 15; (2): CD003934.

[60] Smith CA, Levett KM, Collins CT, Jones L. Massage, reflexology and other manual methods for pain management in labour. *Cochrane Database Syst Rev* (2012) Feb 15; (2): CD009290.

[61] Gitau R, Menson E, Pickles V, et al. Umbilical cortisol levels as an indicator of the fetal stress response to assisted vaginal delivery. *Eur Journal Obstet Gynecol Reprod Biol* (2001) Sept; 98(1): 14-7.

[62] McQuivey RW. Vacuum-assisted delivery: a review. *The Journal of Maternal-Fetal and Neonatal Medicine* (2004) 16: 171-79.

[63] Ali UA, Norwitz ER. Vacuum-assisted vaginal delivery. *Rev Obstet Gynecol* (2009) Winter; 2(1): 5-17.

[64] Bodner-Adler B, Bodner K, Pateisky N, et al. Influence of labor induction on obstetric outcomes in patients with prolonged pregnancy: a comparison between elective labor induction and spontaneous onset of labor beyond term. *Wien Klin Wochenschr* (2005) Apr: 117(7-8): 287-92.

[65] Wang ML, Dorer DJ, Fleming MP, Catlin EA. Clinical outcomes of near-term infants. *Pediatrics* (2004) Aug 1; 114(2): 372-376.

[66] Vardo JH, Thornburg LL, Glantz JC. Maternal and neonatal morbidity among nulliparous women undergoing elective induction of labor. *Journal of Reproductive Medicine* (2011) 56(1-2): 25-30.

[67] Ben-Haroush A, Yogev Y, Bar J, Glickman J, Kaplan H, Hod M. Indicated labor induction with vaginal prostaglandin E2 increases the risk of cesarean section even in multiparous women with no previous cesarean section. *Journal of Perinatal Medicine* (2004) 32(1), 31-36.

[68] Alfirevic Z, Devane D, Gyte GM. Continuous cardiotocography (CTG) as a form of electronic fetal monitoring (EFM) for fetal assessment during labour. *Cochrane Database Syst Rev* (2006) Jul 19; (3): CD006066.

[69] "Screening for Intrapartum Electronic Fetal Monitoring Recommendations." *US Preventive Services Task Force* (1996) <http://www.uspreventiveservicestaskforce.org/uspstf/uspsiefm.htm> (Accessed 13 Feb 2013).

[70] Bakker JJ, Verhoeven CJ, Janssen PF, et al. Outcomes after internal versus external tocodynamometry for monitoring labor. *N Engl J Med* (2010) Jan 28; 362(4): 306-13.

[71] Baenziger O, Stolkin F, Keel M, et al. The influence of the timing of cord clamping on postnatal cerebral oxygenation in preterm neonates: a randomized, controlled trial. *Pediatrics* (2007) Mar; 119(3): 455-9.

[72] Mercer JS, Vohr BR, Oh, W, et al. Delayed cord clamping in very preterm infants reduces the incidence of intraventricular hemorrhage and late-onset sepsis: a randomized controlled trial. *Pediatrics* (2006) Apr; 117(4): 1235-42.

[73] Rabe H, Reynolds G, Diaz-Rossello J. Early versus delayed umbilical cord clamping in preterm infants. *Cochrane Database Syst Rev.* (2004) Oct 18; (4): CD003248.

[74] Chaparro CM, Neufeld LM, Tena Alavez G, et al. Effect of timing of umbilical cord clamping on iron status in Mexican infants: a randomized controlled trial. *Lancet* (2006) Jun 17; 367(9527): 1997-2004.

[75] Frisch M, Lindholm M, Gronbaek M. Male circumcision and sexual function in men and women: a survey-based, cross-sectional study in Denmark. *Int J Epidemiol* (2011) Oct; 40(5): 1367-81.

[76] Fleiss Paul. "The Case Against Circumcision." *Mothering: The Magazine of Natural Family Living.* Winter 1997: 36-45. Reprinted online at <http://www.mothersagainstcirc.org/fleiss.html> (Accessed 13 Dec 2012).

[77] "Reading 'can help reduce stress'," *The Telegraph Online (UK)*, 30 Mar 2009 (The study referred to in the article cited the research of Dr David Lewis, Mindlab International, University of Sussex, 2009).

[78] Berk L, Tan S. "The Laughter - Immune Connection." *The Hospital Clown Newsletter,* 2.2 <http://www.hospitalclown.com/archives/vol-02/vol-2-1and2/vol2-2berk.PDF> (Accessed 15 Dec 2012).

[79] Miller M, Fry WF. The effect of mirthful laughter on the human cardiovascular system. *Medical Hypotheses* (2009) Nov; 73(5): 636.

[80] Kleinke, CL, Peterson TR, Rutledge TR. Effects of self-generated facial expressions on mood. *Journal of Personality and Social Psychology* (1998) 74(1): 272-279.

[81] Zajonc RB, Murphy ST, Inglehart M. "Feeling and facial efference: implications of the vascular theory of emotion." *Psychological Review* (1989) Jul; 96(3): 395-416.

[82] Levine A, Zagoory-Sharon O, Feldman R, Weller A. Oxytocin during pregnancy and early postpartum: individual patterns and maternal-fetal attachment. *Peptides* (2007) Jun; 28(6): 1162-9.

[83] Kisilevsky BS, Hains SM, Lee K, et al. Effects of experience on fetal voice recognition. *Psychol Sci* (2003) May; 14(3): 220-4.

[84] Petitjean C. "Une condition de l'audition foetale: la conduction sonore osseuse. Conséquences cliniques et applications pratiques." Diss. University of Franche-Comté, Besançon, 1989.

[85] May L, Byers-Heinlein K, Werker JF, et al. Language and the newborn brain: does prenatal language experience shape the neonate neural response to speech? *Front Psychol* (2011) Sep 21 2: 222.

[86] Granier-Deferre C, Bassereau S, Ribeiro A, et al. A melodic contour repeatedly experienced by human near-term fetuses elicits a profound cardiac reaction one month after birth. *PLos One* (2011) Feb 23; 6(2): e17304.

[87] King DE, Mainous AG 3rd, Geesey ME, Woolson RF. Dietary magnesium and c-reactive protein levels. *Journal of the American College of Nutrition* (2005) Jun; 24(3): 166-171.

[88] Mauskop A, Altura BM. Role of magnesium in the pathogenesis and treatment of migraines. *Clin Neurosci* (1998); 5(1): 24-7.

[89] Villanueva CM, Gracia-Lavedan E, Ibarluzea J, et al. Exposure to trihalomethanes through different water uses and birth weight, small for gestational age, and preterm delivery in Spain. *Environ Health Perspect* (2011) Dec; 119(12): 1824-1830.

[90] Theoni A, Zech N, Moroder L, Ploner F. Review of 1600 water births. Does water birth increase the risk of neonatal infection? *J Matern Fetal Neonatal Med.* (2005) May; 17(5): 357-61.

[91] Bodner K, Bodner-Adler B, Wierrani F, et al. Effects of water birth on maternal and neonatal outcomes. *Wien Klin Wochesnschr* (2002) Jun 14; 114(10-11): 391-5.

[92] Thoni A, Mussner K, Ploner F. Water birthing: retrospective review of 2625 water births. Contamination of birth pool water and risk of microbial cross-infection. *Minerva Ginecol* (2010) Jun; 62(3): 203-11.

[93] Zhang H, Fan Y, Xia F, et al. Prenatal water deprivation alters brain angiotensin system and dipsogenic changes in the offspring. *Brain Res* (2011) Mar 25; 1382: 128-36.

[94] Melnik B. Milk consumption: aggravating factor of acne and promoter of chronic diseases of Western societies. *Journal of the German Society of Dermatology* (2009) Apr; 7(4): 364-70.

[95] Cordain L, Lindeberg S, Hurtado M, Hill K, Eaton SB, Brand-Miller J. Acne vulgaris. A disease of Western civilization. *Arch Dermatol* (2002); 138: 1584–1590.

[96] Lill C, Loader B, Seemann R, et al. Milk allergy is frequent in patients with chronic sinusitis and nasal polyposis. *Am J Rhinol Allergy* (2011) Nov-Dec; 25(6): e221-4.

[97] Juntti H, Tikkanen S, Kokonen J, Alho OP, Niinimaki A. Cow's milk allergy is associated with recurrent otitis media during childhood. *Acta Otolaryngol* (1999); 119(8): 867-73.

[98] Virtanen SM, Räsänen L, Ylönen K, Aro A, et al. Early introduction of dairy products associated with increased risk of IDDM in Finnish children. *Diabetes* (1993) Dec; 42(12): 1786-1790.

[99] Andıran F, Dayı S, Mete E. Cows milk consumption in constipation and anal fissure in infants and young children. *Journal of Paediatrics and Child Health* (2003) Jul; 39(5): 329–331.

[100] Oliveira MA and Osorio MM. Cow's milk consumption and iron deficiency anemia in children. *J Pediatr* (Rio J) (2005) Sep-Oct; 81(5): 361-7.

[101] Seely S. Diet and coronary disease: a survey of mortality rates and food consumption statistics of 24 countries. *Med Hypotheses* (1981) Jul; 7(7): 907-918.

[102] Feskanich D, Willett WC, Stampfer MJ, Colditz GA. Milk, dietary calcium, and bone fractures in women: a 12-year prospective study. *Am J Publ Health* (1997); 87: 992-7.

[103] Olsen SF, Halldorsson TI, Willett WC, Knudsen VK, Gilman MW, Mikkelsen TB, Olsen J, NUTRIX consortium. Milk consumption during pregnancy is associated with increased infant size at birth: prospective cohort study. *Am J Clin Nutr* (2007) Oct; 86: 1104–10.

[104] Sathyapalan T, Manuchehri AM, Thatcher NJ, et al. The effect of soy phytoestrogen supplementation on thyroid status and cardiovascular risk markers in patients with subclinical hypothyroidism: a randomized, double-blind, crossover study. *J Clin Endocrinol Metab.* (2011) May; 96(5): 1442-9.

[105] Touillaud MS, Pillow PC, Jakovljevic J, et al. Effect of dietary intake of phytoestrogens on estrogen receptor status in premenopausal women with breast cancer. *Nutr Cancer.* (2005) 51(2): 162-9.

[106] Hwang BF, Jaakkola JJ, Guo HR. Water disinfection by-products and the risk of specific birth defects: a population-based cross-sectional study in Taiwan. *Environ Health* (2008); Jun 2; 7:23.

[107] Madhusudhan N, Basha PM, Rai P, Ahmed F, Prasad GR. Effect of maternal fluoride exposure on developing CNS of rats: protective role of Aloe vera, Curuma longa and Ocimum sanctum. *Indian J Exp Biol* (2010) Aug; 48(8): 830-6.

[108] Zeng Q, Cui YS, Zhang L, et al. Studies of fluoride on the thyroid cell apoptosis and mechanism. *Zhonghua Yu Fang Yi Xue Za Zhi* (2012) Mar; 46(3): 233-6.

[109] He LF, Chen JG. DNA damage, apoptosis and cell cycle changes induced by fluoride in rat oral mucosal cells and hepatocytes. *World J Gastroenterol* (2006) Feb 21; 12(7): 1144-8.

[110] Luke J. "The Effect of Fluoride on the Physiology of the Pineal Gland." Ph.D Diss. University of Surrey, Guildford, 1997. <http://www.slweb.org/luke-1997.html> (Accessed 17 Jan 2012).

[111] National Research Council. *Fluoride in Drinking Water: A Scientific Review of EPA's Standards*. Washington DC: National Academies Press, 2006.

[112] Rosborg I, Nihlgard B, and Gerhardsson L. Inorganic constituents of well water in one acid and one alkaline area of south Sweden. *Water Air Soul Pollution* (2003) 142: 261-277.

[113] Sánchez-Villegas A, Toledo E, de Irala J, et al. Fast-food and commercial baked goods consumption and the risk of depression. *Public Health Nutrition* (2012) Mar; 15 (3): 424-32.

[114] Appleton N. Lick the Sugar Habit (1996) Avery, 2nd Ed. 272 pp.

[115] Huber D. "Letter from Dr. Huber to European Commission," *Farm & Ranch Freedom Alliance*. Mar 2011. <http://farmandranchfreedom.org/Huber-European-letter> (Accessed 12 Jan 2012).

[116] Netherwood, T. Assessing the survival of transgenic plant DNA in the human gastrointestinal tract. *Nature Biotechnology* (2004) 22: 204-209.

[117] Aris A, Leblanc S. Maternal and fetal exposure associated to genetically modified foods in Eastern townships of Canada. *Reprod Toxicol* (2011) May; 31 (4): 528-33.

[118] Seralini GE, Clair E, Mesnage R, et al. Long term toxicity of a Roundup herbicide and a Roundup-tolerant genetically modified maize. *Food and Chemical Toxicity* (2012) Nov; 50(11): 4221-31.

[119] Daniel, Kaayla T. *The Whole Soy Story*. Washington, DC: New Trends Publishing Inc, 2005.

[120] Foster WG, Chan S, Platt L, Hughes CL Jr. Detection of phytoestrogens in samples of second trimester human amniotic fluid. *Toxicology Letters* (2002) Mar 28; 129(3): 199-205.

[121] Rust S and Kissinger M. "BPA leaches from 'safe' products." *Journal Sentinel Online* 15 Nov 2008. <http://www.jsonline.com/watchdog/watchdogreports/34532034.html> (Accessed 17 Jan 2012).

[122] Kopp, William, "Microwave Madness: The Effects of Microwave Apparatus on Food and Humans," *Perceptions* (1996) May/June: 30-3.

[123] Quan R, Yang C, Rubinstein S, et al. Effects of microwave radiation on anti-infective factors in human milk. *Pediatrics* (1992) Apr; 89 (4 part I): 667-9.

[124] Arielle Reynolds, "Microwaved Water,"
http://rense.com/general70/microwaved.htm

[125] http://nutritiondata.self.com/

[126] Leung BM, Kaplan BJ. Perinatal depression: prevalence, risks, and the nutrition link—a review of the literature. *J Am Diet Assoc* (2009) Sep; 109(9): 1566-75. doi: 10.1016/j.jada.2009.06.368.

[127] Coletta JM, Bell SJ, Roman AS. Omega-3 fatty acids and pregnancy. *Rev Obstet Gynecol* (2010) Fall; 3(4): 163-171.

[128] Aben A, Danckaerts M. Omega-3 and omega-6 fatty acids in the treatment of children and adolescents with ADHD. *Tijdschr Psychiatr* (2010) 52(2): 89-97.

[129] "Omega-3 fatty acids." University of Maryland Medical Center, n.d. <http://www.umm.edu/altmed/articles/omega-3-000316.htm> (Accessed 16 Feb 2013).

[130] Yashodhara BM. Omega-3 fatty acids: a comprehensive review of their role in health and disease. *Postgrad Med J* (2009) 85(1000): 84-90.

[131] Andrade SE, Gurwitz JH, Davis RL, Chan A, Finkelstein JA, Fortman K, et al. Prescription drug use in pregnancy. *Am J Obstet Gynecol* (2004) 191(2): 398–407.

[132] Beddoe AE, et al. The effects of mindfulness-based yoga during pregnancy on maternal psychological and physical distress. *J Obstet Gynecol Neonatal Nurs* (2009) May-Jun; 38(3): 310-9.

[133] Beddoe AE, Lee KA. Mind-body interventions during pregnancy. *J Obstet Gynecol Neonatal Nurs* (2008) Mar-Apr; 37(2): 165-75.

[134] Csoka AB, Szyf M. Epigenetic side-effects of common pharmaceuticals: a potential new field in medicine and pharmacology. *Med Hypotheses* (2009) 73: 770–780.

[135] Haire, Doris. "FDA approved obstetrics drugs: their effects on mother and baby." National Women's Health Alliance (2001) <http://www.aimsusa.org/obstetricdrugs.htm> (Accessed 17 April 2012).

[136] Andrade SE, Gurwitz JH, Davis RL, et al. Prescription drug use in pregnancy. *Am J Obstet Gynecol* (2004) Aug; 191(2): 398-407.

[137] Nakhai-Pour HR, Broy P, Berard A. Use of antidepressants during pregnancy and the risk of spontaneous abortion. *CMAJ* (2010) Jul; 182(10): 1031-1037.

[138] Wen SW, Yang Q, Garner P, Fraser W, et al. Selective serotonin reuptake inhibitors (SSRIS) and adverse pregnancy outcomes. *Am J Obstet Gyn* (2005) Dec; 193(6). doi: 10.1016/j.ajog.2005.10.095.

[139] Lund N, Pedersen LH, Henriksen TB. Selective serotonin reuptake inhibitor exposure in utero and pregnancy outcomes. *Arch Pediatr Adolesc Med* (2009) Oct; 163(10): 949-54.

[140] Wurst KE, Poole C, Ephross SA, Olshan AF. First trimester paroxetine use and the prevalence of congenital, specifically cardiac, defects: a meta-analysis of epidemiological studies. *Birth Defects Research Part A: Clinical and Molecular Teratology* (2010) Mar; 88(3): 159-70.

[141] Chambers CD, Hernandez-Diaz S, Van Marter LJ, et al. Selective serotonin-reuptake inhibitors and risk of persistent pulmonary hypertension of the newborn. *N Engl J Med* (2006) 354(6): 579-87.

[142] Croen LA, Grether JK, Yoshida CK, Odouli R, Hendrick V. Antidepressant use during pregnancy and childhood autism spectrum disorders. *Arch Gen Psychiatry* (2011) Nov; 68(11): 1104-12.

[143] Pedersen LH, Henriksen TB, Vestergaard M, Olsen J, Bech B. Selective serotonin reuptake inhibitors in pregnancy and congenital malformations: population based cohort study. *BMJ* (2009) Sep; 339: b3569.

[144] Alwan S, Reefhuis J, Rasmussen SA, et al. Use of selective serotonin-reuptake inhibitors in pregnancy and the risk of birth defects. *NEngl J Med* (2007) Jun 28; 356(26): 2684-92.

[145] Are antidepressants safe in pregnancy? A focus on SSRIs. *Therapeutics Letter* (2010) Jan/Feb 76. <http://www.ti.ubc.ca/letter76> (Accessed 9 Dec 2011).

[146] Kirsch I, Deacon BJ, Huedo-Medina TB, et al. Initial severity and antidepressant benefits: a meta-analysis of data submitted to the Food and Drug Administration. *PLoS Med* (2008) 5(2): e45.

[147] Buscicchio G, Piemontese M, Gentilucci L, Ferretti F, Tranquilli AL. The effects of maternal caffeine and chocolate intake on fetal heart rate. *J Matern Fetal Neonatal Med* (2012) May; 25(5): 528-30.

[148] Wendler CC, Busovsky-McNeal M, Ghatpande S, Kalinowski A, Russell KS, Rivkees SA. Embryonic caffeine exposure induces adverse effects in adulthood. *FASEB J* (2009) April; 23(4): 1272-1278.

[149] Yazdani M, Joseph F Jr, Grant S, Hartman AD, Nakamoto T. Various levels of maternal caffeine ingestion during gestation affects biochemical parameters of fetal rat brain differently. *Dev Pharmacol Ther* (1990); 14(1): 52-61.

[150] Tan Y, Liu J, Deng Y, et al. Caffeine-induced fetal rat over-exposure to maternal glucocorticoid and histone methylation of liver IGF-1 might cause skeletal growth retardation. *Toxicol Lett* (2012) Nov 15; 214(3): 279-87.

[151] Xu D, Zhang B, Liang G, Ping J, Kou H, et al. Caffeine-induced activated glucocorticoid metabolism in the hippocampus causes hypothalamic-pituitary-adrenal axis inhibition in fetal rats. *PLoS One* (2012); 7(9): e44497. doi: 10.1371/journal.pone.0044497.

[152] Seifert SM, Schaechter JL, Hershorin ER, Lipshultz SE. Health effects of energy drinks on children, adolescents, and young adults. *Pediatrics* (2011) March; 127(3): 511-528.

[153] Weng X, Odouli R, Li DK. Maternal caffeine consumption during pregnancy and the risk of miscarriage: a prospective cohort study. *Am J Obstet Gynecol* (2008) Mar; 198(3): 279.e1-279.e8.

[154] Dahl RE, Scher MS, Williamson DE, Robles N, Day N. A longitudinal study of prenatal marijuana use. Effects on sleep and arousal at age 3 years. *Arch Pediatr Adolesc Med* (1995) Feb; 149(2): 145-50.

[155] Goldschmidt L, Day NL, Richardson GA. Effects of prenatal marijuana exposure on child behavior problems at age 10. *Neurotoxicol Teratol* (2000) May-Jun; 22(3): 325-36.

[156] Gray KA, Day NL, Leech S, Richardson GA. Prenatal marijuana exposure: effect on child depressive symptoms at tens years of age. *Neurotoxicol Teratol* (2005) May-Jun; 27(3): 439-48.

[157] Abel EL. Prenatal effects of alcohol. *Drug Alcohol Depend* (1984) Sep; 14(1): 1-10.

[158] Office on Smoking and Health (US). *Women and Smoking: A Report of the Surgeon General.* Atlanta (GA): Centers for Disease Control and Prevention (US); 2001 Mar. Chapter 3. Health Consequences of Tobacco Use Among Women.

[159] U.S. Department of Health and Human Services. *The Health Consequences of Smoking: Nicotine Addiction: A Report of the Surgeon General.* Rockville, Maryland: U.S. Department of Health and Human Services, Public Health Service, Centers for Disease Control, Center for Health Promotion and Education, Office on Smoking and Health, 1988.

[160] U.S. Department of Health and Human Services. *Reducing the Health Consequences of Smoking: 25 years of progress: A Report of the Surgeon General.* Rockville, Maryland: U.S. Department of Health and Human Services, Public Health Service, Centers for Disease Control, Center for Chronic Disease Prevention and Health Promotion, Office on Smoking and Health, 1989.

[161] U.S. Department of Health and Human Services. *The Health Consequences of Smoking for Women: A report of the Surgeon General.* Rockville, Maryland: U.S. Department of Health and Human Services, Public Health Service, Office of the Assistant Secretary for Health, Office on Smoking and Health, 1980.

[162] Weitzman M, Gortmaker S, Sobol A. Maternal smoking and behaviour problems of children. *Pediatrics* (1992) 90: 342-349.

[163] California Environmental Protection Agency. *Health Effects of Exposure to Environmental Tobacco Smoke: Final Report.* Sacramento: California Environmental Protection Agency, Office of Environmental Health Hazard Assessment, 1997.

[164] Ashford KB, et al. The effects of prenatal secondhand smoke exposure on preterm birth and neonatal outcomes. *J Obstet Gynecol Neonatal Nurs* (2010) Sep-Oct; 39(5): 525-35.

[165] De Iuliis GN, Newey RJ, King BV, Aitken RJ. Mobile phone radiation induces oxygen species production and DNA damage in human spermatozoa in vitro. *PLoS One* (2009) Jul 31; 4(7): e6446.

[166] Hardell L, Sage C. Biological effects from electromagnetic field exposure and public exposure standards. *Biomed Pharmacother* (2008) Feb; 62(2): 104-9.

[167] Owen N, Bauman A, Brown W. Too much sitting: a novel and important predictor of chronic disease risk? *Br J Sports Med* (2009) 43: 81-83.

[168] "Physiologists And Microbiologists Find Link Between Sitting And Poor Health." *Sciencedaily.com.* Science Daily, 1 June 2008. <http://www.sciencedaily.com/videos/2008/0610-stand_up_for_your_health.htm> (Accessed 15 Jan 2012).

[169] Hartikainen AL, Sorri M, Anttonen H, Tuimala R, Laara E. Effect of occupational noise on the course and outcome of pregnancy. *Scand J Work Environ Health* (1994) 20:444-450.

[170] Knipschild P, Meijer H, Sallé H. Aircraft noise and birth weight. *International Archives of Occupational and Environmental Health* (1981) 48: 131-136.

[171] Lalande NM, Hetu R, Lambert J. Is occupational noise exposure during pregnancy a risk factor of damage to the auditory system of the fetus? *Am J Ind Med* (1986) 10:427-435.

[172] Schneider ML. Prenatal stress exposure alters postnatal behavioral expression under conditions of novelty challenge in rhesus monkey infants. *Developmental Psychobiology* (1992) 25(7): 529-540.

[173] Clarke S, Soto A, Bergholz T, Schneider ML. Maternal gestational stress alters adaptive and social behavior in adolescent rhesus monkey offspring. *Infant Behavior and Development* (1996) 19.4: 451–461.

[174] Khattak S, Moghtader G, McMartin K, Barrera M, Kennedy D, Koren G. Pregnancy outcome following gestational exposure to organic solvents: a prospective, controlled study. *JAMA* (1999) 281, 1106-1109.

[175] Silver, Curtis. "Neurocinema Aims to Change the Way Movies are Made," *Wired.com.* Wired Magazine, 23 Sept 2009. <www.wired.com/geekdad/2009/09/neurocinema-aims-to-change-the-way-movies-are-made> (Accessed 11 Dec 2011).

[176] Wager TD, Barrett LF, Bliss-Moreau E, Lindquist K, et al. The neuroimaging of emotion. In Lewis M, Haviland-Jones JM, and Barrett LF (Eds.), *Handbook of Emotions* (3rd ed), New York: Guilford Press (2010).

[177] Maren, S. Neurobiology of pavlovian fear conditioning. *Annual Revue of Neuroscience* (2001) Vol. 24: 897–931.

[178] "The Global Forest." Inter. Anna Maria Tremonti. Guest Diana Beresford-Kroeger. *The Current.* CBC. 18 May 2010. Radio.

[179] Goel N, Etwaroo GR. Bright light, negative air ions and auditory stimuli produce rapid mood changes in student population: a placebo-controlled study. *Psychol Med* (2006) Sep; 36 (9): 1253-63.

[180] Goel N, Terman M, Terman JS, Macchi MM, Stewart JW. Controlled trial of bright light and negative air ions for chronic depression, *Psychol Med* (2005) Jul; 35(7): 945-55.

[181] Morton LL, Kershner JR. Negative air ionization improves memory and attention in learning-disabled and mentally retarded children. *J Abnorm Child Psychol* (1994) Jun; 12(2): 353-65.

[182] Perrera FP, Li Z, Whyatt R, Hoepner L, Wang S, Camann D, Rauh V. Prenatal airborne polycyclic aromatic hydrocarbon exposure and child IQ at age 5 years. *Pediatrics* (2009) Aug 124(2): e195-202.

[183] Bolton JL, Smith SH, Huff NC, et al. Prenatal air pollution exposure induces neuroinflammation and predisposes offspring to weight gain in adulthood in a sex-specific manner. *FASEB J* (2012) Nov; 26(11): 4743-54.

[184] Rundle A, Hoepner L, Hassoun A, et al. Association of childhood obesity with maternal exposure to ambient air polycyclic aromatic hydrocarbons during pregnancy. *Am J of Epidemiol* (2012) Jun 1; 175(11): 1163-72.

[185] Perera FP, Wang S, Vishnevetsky J, et al. Polycyclic aromatic hydrocarbons-aromatic DNA adducts in cord blood and behavior scores in New York city children. *Environ Health Perspect* (2011) Aug; 119(8): 1176-81.

[186] Padula AM, Humblet O, Mortimer K, Lurmann F, Tager I. "Exposure To Air Pollution During Pregnancy And Pulmonary Function Growth In The FACES LiTE Cohort." American Thoracic Society 2012 International Conference (Session A49, Sunday, May 20, 2012: 8:15 a.m. - 4:30 p.m., Area A, Moscone Center; Abstract 31611).

[187] Ruchat SM, et al. Walking program of low or vigorous intensity during pregnancy confers an aerobic benefit. *Int J Sports Med* (2012) Apr 17.

[188] Van Den Berg AE, Custers MH. Gardening promotes neuroendocrine and affective restoration from stress. *J Health Psychol* (2011) Jan; 16(1): 3-11.

[189] Waldie KE, Poulton R, Kirk IJ, Silva PA. The effects of pre- and post-natal sunlight exposure on human growth: evidence from the Southern Hemisphere. *Early Human Dev* (2000) Nov; 60(1): 35-42.

[190] Sayers A, Tobias JH. Estimated maternal ultraviolet B exposure levels in pregnancy influence skeletal development of the child. *J Clin Endocrinol Metab* (2009) Mar; 94(3): 765-71.

[191] Montagu, Ashley. *Touching: The Human Significance of the Skin*. New York: Harper, 1986.

[192] Gottlieb DJ, Punjabi NM, Newman AB, et al. Association of sleep time with diabetes mellitus and impaired glucose tolerance. *Arch. Intern. Med* (2005) 165 (8): 863–7.

[193] Kripke DF, Langer RD, Kline LE. Hypnotics' association with mortality or cancer: a matched cohort study. *BMJ Open* (2012) 2:1 e000850.

[194] Vgontzas An, et al. Chronic insomnia is associated with nyctohemeral activation of the hypothalamic-pituitary-adrenal axis: clinical implications. *Journal of Clinical Endocrinology and Metabolism* (2001) Aug; 86(8): 3787-3794.

[195] Chang MY, Chen CH, Huang KF. Effects of music therapy on psychological health of women during pregnancy. *J Clin Nurs* (2008) Oct; 17(19): 2580-7.

[196] Harmat L, Takács J, Bódizs R. Music improves sleep quality in students. *Journal of Advanced Nursing* (2008) May; 62(3): 327-35.

[197] Ventura T, Gomes MC, Carreira T. Cortisol and anxiety response to a relaxing intervention on pregnant women awaiting amniocentesis. *Psychoneuroendocrinology* (2012) Jan; 37(1): 148-56.

[198] Arya R, Chansoria M, Konanki R, Tiwari DK. Maternal music exposure during pregnancy influences neonatal behaviour: an open-label randomized control trial. *Int J Pediatrics* (2012) 2012: 901812. Epub 2012 Feb 14.

[199] Kim H, Lee MH, et al. Influence of prenatal noise and music on the spatial memory and neurogenesis in the hippocampus of developing rats. *Brain Dev* (2006) Mar; 28(2): 109-14.

[200] Kauser H, Roy S, Pal A, et al. Prenatal complex rhythmic music sound stimulation facilitates postnatal spatial learning but transiently impairs memory in the domestic chick. *Dev Neurosci* (2011) 33(1): 48-56.

[201] Malinova M, Malinolva M. Effect of music on fetal behaviour. *Akush Gineko (Sophia)* (2004); 43 Suppl 4:25-8.

[202] Dempsey JC, Butler CL, Sorensen TK, Lee IM, Thompson ML, Miller RS. A case-control study of maternal recreational physical activity and risk of gestational diabetes mellitus. *Diabetes Res Clin Pract* (2004) 66(2):203–15.

[203] Sorensen TK, Williams MA, Lee IM, Dashow EE, Thompson ML, Luthy DA. Recreational physical activity during pregnancy and risk of preeclampsia. *Hypertension* (2003) 41: 1273–80.

[204] Magnus P, Trogstad L, Owe KM, Olsen SF, Nystad W. Recreational physical activity and the risk of preeclampsia: a prospective cohort of Norwegian women. *American Journal of Epidemiology* (2008) 168: 952–957.

[205] Yeo S. Prenatal stretching exercise and autonomic responses: preliminary data and a model for reducing preeclampsia. *Journal Nurs Scholarsh* (2010) June 1; 42(2): 113-121.

[206] Lu WA, Kuo CD. The effect of Tai Chi Chuan on the autonomic nervous modulation in older persons. *Medicine & Science in Sports & Exercise* (2003) 35:1972–1976.

[207] Pukui, MK and Elbert, SH. *Hawaiian Dictionary*. University of Hawai'i Press (2003).

[208] Ullrich PM, Lutgendorf SK. Journaling about stressful events: effects of cognitive processing and emotional expression. *Annals of Behavioral Medicine* (2002) 24:244–250.

[209] Smith BW, Shelley BM, Dalen J, Wiggens K, Tooley E, Bernard J. A pilot study comparing the effects of mindfulness-based and cognitive –behavioral stress reduction. *J Altern Complement Med* (2008) Apr; 14(3): 251-8.

[210] Verny, T. *Tomorrow's Baby: The Art and Science of Parenting from Conception Through Infancy*. New York: Simon and Schuster (2002).

[211] Jallo N, Bourguignon C, Taylor AG, Utz SW. Stress management during pregnancy: designing and evaluating a mind-body intervention. *Fam Community Health* (2008) Jul-Sep; 31(3): 190-2-3.

[212] Vieten C, Astin J. Effects of a mindfulness-based intervention during pregnancy on prenatal stress and mood: results of a pilot study. *Arch Womens Mental Health* (2008) 11(1): 67-74.

Printed in Great Britain
by Amazon